Diabetes
for **Nurses**

Second Edition

Diabetes for Nurses

SECOND EDITION

Lynne Jerreat

BSc (Hons), RGN, FETC

Diabetes Specialist Nurse, Queen Elizabeth Hospital, London

With a contribution from

Cathy Parker

MSc, BEd (Hons), RGN, RM, RHV, RNT

Senior Lecturer, University of Surrey and
the Royal College of Nursing, London

Whurr Publishers Ltd
London and Philadelphia

© 2003 Whurr Publishers Ltd
First Edition published 1999
Second Edition published 2003 by
Whurr Publishers Ltd
19b Compton Terrace
London N1 2UN England and
325 Chestnut Street Philadelphia PA 19106, USA

Reprinted 2004

British Library Cataloguing in Publication Data
A catalogue record for this book is available from the
British Library.

ISBN 1 86156 295 0

Printed and bound in the UK
by Athenaeum Press Limited, Gateshead, Tyne & Wear.

Contents

Abbreviations

ACE	angiotensin-converting enzyme
ADA	American Diabetes Association
AIDS	Acquired Immune Deficiency Syndrome
BD	Becton Dickinson
BDA	British Diabetic Association
BG	blood glucose
BMI	body mass index
BP	blood pressure
BSE	bovine spongiform encephalopathy
CAPD	continuous ambulatory peritoneal dialysis
CHO	carbohydrate
CSAG	Clinical Standards Advisory Group
CSII	continuous subcutaneous infusion of insulin
CT	computed tomography
DAFNE	dose adjustment for normal eating
DCCT	Diabetes Control and Complications Trial
DDCC	Diabetes Day Care Centres
DKA	diabetic ketoacidosis
DoH	Department of Health
DSM	diabetes specialist midwife
DSN	diabetes specialist nurse
DSS	Department of Social Services
DVLA	Driver and Vehicle Licensing Agency
ECG	electrocardiogram
ESRF	end-stage renal failure
FPG	fasting plasma glucose
GKI	glucose potassium regime
GMSC	General Medical Services Committee
GP	general practitioner
GTT	glucose tolerance test
HbA1	glycated haemoglobin
HbA1$_c$	glycated haemoglobin
HBGM	home blood glucose monitoring

HBM	Health Belief Model
HDL	high-density lipoprotein
HGV	heavy goods vehicle
HLA	human leucocyte antigen
HNF	hepatic nuclear factor
HONK	hyper-osmolar non-ketotic syndrome
HUT	home urine testing
ID	identification
IFG	impaired fasting glucose
IGT	impaired glucose tolerance
IRMA	intra-retinal microvascular anomalies
ITD	insulin-treated diabetes
IVU	intravenous urogram
LDL	low-density lipoprotein
LDSAGs	Local Diabetes Service Advisory Groups
MODY	maturity-onset diabetes of the young
MUSE	medicated urethral system for erection
NEFA	non-esterified fatty acids
NG	nasogastric
NHS	National Health Service
OGTT	oral glucose tolerance test
PCT	Primary Care Trust
PMS	Personal Medical Services
PSV	public service vehicle
PVD	peripheral vascular disease
RBG	random blood glucose
RCN	Royal College of Nursing
RDS	respiratory distress syndrome
UKPDS	United Kingdom Prospective Diabetes Study
VLDL	very-low-density lipoprotein
WHO	World Health Organisation

Preface

This book is intended to be a comprehensive guide to diabetes for nurses in Britain. It is particularly aimed at diploma and degree-level students, 'new' Practice Nurses and 'new' Diabetes Specialist Nurses. It is hoped that other health care workers may also find it useful.

Diabetes is addressed both as a biochemical disease and a psychosocial problem. The management of diabetes on a day-to-day basis is the patients' domain; they become the experts. Changing life events such as illness, surgery, pregnancy or bereavement can disrupt equilibrium. Blood glucose control and emotional adjustment to diabetes are therefore potentially unstable. Advice and support may be required at these times.

The 'diabetic' can be seen as threatening to nurses; such individuals may appear knowledgeable, sometimes leading to their being 'left to it'. Some patients may be critical; they may know if blood glucose measurements are performed incorrectly, and the time tablets or insulin should be given in relation to meals. Others may be 'out of date' or having problems which could benefit from sensitive education by the nurse.

The aim of the book is to provide research-based information about diabetes and suggestions for problem-solving and planning care. The main objectives are: that diabetes management will not be seen merely in terms of blood glucose; that those with diabetes will be treated as individuals with differing needs, health care beliefs and lifestyles; and that the importance of a team approach, with the patient as central to the team, will be realized.

I would like to thank Dr Philip Marsden for all his help and encouragement, and Denise Murphy for her help with the illustrations.

Introduction

Four per cent of the world's population aged 20 years and above were estimated to have diabetes in 1995 (135 million), and this number is likely to rise to 5.4 per cent (300 million) by 2025 (King et al., 1998). Diabetes can have a major impact on the physical, psychological, social and economic health of individuals, and can lead to complications such as cardiovascular disease, blindness, renal failure and amputation. The National Service Framework Standards (NSF) were published by the government in December 2001, and the implementation strategy was published in January 2003. The NSF is discussed in full by Cathy Parker in Chapter 8, and the standard(s) that I consider most relevant to each chapter are contained in a box at the end of the chapter. It is hoped that this will help us to reflect on how we can best help to meet the new standards.

The book is designed so that each chapter is self-contained and can be read in isolation, although each builds on information from previous chapters. The chapters are organized systematically, beginning with what diabetes is and ending with the organization of diabetes care in the community. Chapters are cross-referenced where appropriate. A list of references is provided at the end of each chapter and case-studies are used throughout the book. Learning outcomes are identified for each chapter and questions at the end of each chapter help readers to assess their knowledge. Answers to these questions are given at the end of the book. The intention of the book in its entirety is to look at the care of the person with diabetes through a holistic approach.

The philosophy of the book is based on that of the Diabetes Day Care Centre in which I work. The person with diabetes is approached as an individual. We accept that each person has his or her own value system, set of health care beliefs, level of understanding and experience which is unique to that person. The aims and objectives of care and the resulting educational programmes are tailored to the needs of the individual. Information is given in small manageable amounts, and knowledge obtained is revised and built upon.

We aim to become partners in care with patients, enabling them to make informed decisions and promoting independence. The information and care given are research and theoretically based and are evaluated. Diabetes care is approached from a team perspective. The person with diabetes has access to a range of health care professionals and a 'patient helper', who communicate with one another, share ideas, support and educate one another. This attempts to ensure that the information and advice given to patients is complementary rather than contradictory and confusing.

The person with diabetes is referred to as a patient rather than a client, user or consumer in the book. All of these terms are problematic. 'Patient' implies a passive individual to whom the health professional does things. 'Consumer' or 'customer' implies that payment is required; this term is still unacceptable to some in a health service which has traditionally been free at the point of delivery. 'User' carries undertones of drug dependency, and the term 'client' is commonly used to describe those attending hairdressing salons or estate agents. I personally feel that client, consumer or user do not adequately describe the depth of the relationship between the nurse and the person with a chronic disease.

The book is divided into three sections. The first section introduces diabetes and addresses fundamental questions. These include: the definition of diabetes, the altered physiology, the symptoms, the diagnosis, the types of diabetes and the treatments available. The side-effects of the various treatments and the complications of the disease are also discussed. The Diabetes Control and Complications Trial (DCCT), the United Kingdom Prospective Diabetes Study (UKPDS) and the St Vincent's Declaration are referred to in the chapter that discusses diabetic complications.

Section two addresses the practice of patient education and clinical management of diabetes. The multidisciplinary team approach to diabetes is fundamental to diabetes management and this approach runs through this section. Subjects such as monitoring of blood glucose levels and urine testing, the initiation, drawing up, administration and adjustments of insulin, foot care, the role of Diabetes UK, driving and employment are included. The adjustment of insulin for changes in lifestyle, intercurrent illness, travel involving time-zone changes, exercise and clinical investigations are allowed an entire chapter. The care of special groups of people with diabetes – the elderly, the pregnant, those in hospital and those from ethnic minority groups – has been allocated a specific chapter.

Section three aims to put diabetes care into context. It attempts to examine the broader issues involved in diabetes care and hopes to prevent diabetes being seen in a vacuum. Psychological issues – grief and mourning, the adaptation to lifestyle changes, health care beliefs, needle phobias and the psychological support needed – are discussed. The expansion of primary care involvement in the management of diabetes is discussed by Cathy Parker, an experienced practitioner and lecturer in diabetes care.

Reference

King H, Aubert RE, Herman WH (1998) Global burden of diabetes, 1995–2025: prevalence, numerical estimates and projections. Diabetes Care 21: 1414–31.

SECTION ONE
INTRODUCTION TO DIABETES

Chapter 1
The diagnosis and classification of diabetes mellitus

In this chapter I shall define what diabetes is and how to diagnose it. The various types of diabetes mellitus will be classified and the differential diagnosis of Type 1 diabetes (previously called insulin-dependent diabetes) and Type 2 diabetes (previously called non-insulin-dependent diabetes) will be addressed. Maturity-onset diabetes of the young (MODY) and impaired glucose tolerance will also be discussed briefly.

Learning Outcomes

After reading this chapter you should be able to:

(1) identify the symptoms of diabetes and provide an explanation of why they occur
(2) demonstrate confidence in the use of the World Health Organisation (WHO) diagnostic criteria for diabetes
(3) distinguish whether a patient with newly diagnosed diabetes has Type 1 or Type 2 diabetes.

What is Diabetes Mellitus?

Diabetes mellitus is a metabolic disorder in which the body has a deficiency of, and/or a resistance to, insulin.

What is insulin and how does it work?

Insulin is a hormone produced by the beta cells of the islets of Langerhans in the pancreas. The function of insulin is to regulate blood glucose levels. As blood glucose levels rise after a carbohydrate-containing meal, insulin is produced which allows surplus glucose to be stored in the liver and muscle as glycogen. If food is unavailable the blood glucose level falls, insulin production falls and liver glycogen is broken down into glucose. This process is called glycogenolysis.

Another process, gluconeogenesis, begins when insulin levels are low. Protein and fat are broken down and used by the liver to synthesize glucose.

Insulin also encourages the storage of surplus carbohydrate as fat. Lack of insulin in response to less food allows fat to be broken down and used to provide energy. The processes involved are lipolysis which breaks down triglycerides and converts glycerol to glucose, and ketogenesis in which ketones are synthesized in the liver.

Insulin production indicates that food and energy are in good supply and dietary protein can be used to build and repair tissues. If insulin, and therefore energy, is in short supply gluconeogenesis uses protein to synthesize glucose and mobilizes protein from the tissues to provide energy.

In health this system is so efficient that blood glucose levels vary very little. They tend to remain stable at around 3–8 mmol/L.

What happens in diabetes?

Lack of insulin or a resistance to insulin has major metabolic effects. Carbohydrate cannot be utilized effectively and surplus glucose cannot be stored in the liver. The glucose level in the blood increases but the cells of the body are in fact deprived of glucose and energy. Shortage of insulin leads to glycogen, fat and protein being broken down into glucose. This glucose cannot be utilized by the body without insulin, making the blood glucose level even higher.

Hyperglycaemia leads to glucose spilling over into the urine, which leads to a marked osmotic diuresis. The patient commonly experiences polyuria and nocturia and therefore loses excessive amounts of water, sodium and potassium in the urine. This increased diuresis leads to increased thirst. The loss of glucose in the urine may lead to weight loss and tiredness. The presence of glucose in the urine encourages infection with yeasts causing irritation of the vulva or penis.

Glucose concentration may temporarily affect the lens of the eye (not to be confused with diabetic retinopathy, see p. 66). The lens of the eye becomes swollen when blood glucose is high and this leads to blurred vision. A person with newly diagnosed diabetes should wait a few months after diabetes is controlled before visiting the optician for new glasses as eyesight usually returns to 'normal'. The breakdown of muscle protein can lead to weakness and muscle wasting. Breakdown of fat can lead to further weight loss. The presenting symptoms of diabetes vary enormously depending on the degree of insulin deficiency. If there is no available insulin, symptoms will be severe and large quantities of ketones will be present in the urine owing to the reliance of the body on fat stores for energy. This can lead to acidosis and death.

The Diagnosis of Diabetes

There are psychological, social and economic implications for the person diagnosed with diabetes. The diagnosis must therefore be accurate. The World Health Organisation (WHO, 1980, 1985, 1999) established diagnostic criteria which are used in Britain.

There has been some disagreement between the American Diabetes Association (ADA) Expert Committee on the Diagnosis and Classification of Diabetes Mellitus (1997) and the World Health Organisation (WHO) regarding the diagnosis and classification of diabetes. This has resulted in the amended diagnostic criteria of the WHO (1999) and the adoption of the terms Type 1 and Type 2 diabetes. Type 1 describes the cause of the disease; beta cell destruction leading to insulin deficiency. Type 2 diabetes ranges from insulin resistance with relative insulin deficiency to secretory defect with or without insulin resistance.

Box 1.1: The criteria for the diagnosis of diabetes (WHO, 1999)

1.

• Symptoms of diabetes

PLUS

• A random venous plasma glucose concentration of ≥ 11.1 mmol/L

or

• A fasting plasma glucose concentration of ≥ 7.0 mmol/L
    (whole blood ≥ 6.1 mmol/L)

or

2.
• A 2-hour plasma glucose concentration of ≥ 11.1 mmol/L 2 hours
    after 75g anhydrous glucose in an oral glucose tolerance test (OGTT).

In the absence of diabetes symptoms, diagnosis should **not** be made on a single glucose determination. At least one other laboratory plasma venous determination is required on another day with a value in the diabetic range. This can be fasting, a random sample or from the 2-hour post glucose load. If the fasting or random levels are not diagnostic, the 2-hour post glucose value should be used.

The WHO (1999) recommends that ideally both the 2-hour and the fasting value should be used. These recommendations contrast with those of the ADA Expert Committee (1997) which give priority to the fasting plasma glucose. The WHO claim that it has been shown that some of the individuals identified by the new fasting values differ from those identified by 2-hour post glucose challenge values. These include the elderly and those with less obesity, such as many Asian populations. In contrast, middle-aged, more obese patients are likely to have diagnostic fasting values.

The presence of glucose in the urine is not adequate to diagnose diabetes. Indeed, glycosuria can be present in those without diabetes who have a low renal threshold. A blood glucose meter on the ward or at the GP surgery is inadequate to confirm or eliminate diabetes. A laboratory blood glucose estimation is necessary. HbA1$_c$ and fructosamine estimations are also unreliable and should not be used to diagnose diabetes. Anaemia, haemoglobinopathies and uraemia may all influence their reliability.

The World Health Organisation published a revised 'Definition, Diagnosis and Classification of Diabetes Mellitus and its Complications' in 1999. Diabetes UK (previously the BDA) recommended that it be adopted in Britain from 1 June 2000.

The biggest change from the previous criteria was that the cut-off point for diagnosis of diabetes using a fasting plasma glucose was reduced from 7.8 mmol/L to 7.0 mmol/L. This reduction is based on research findings that demonstrated microvascular abnormalities in patients with fasting glycaemia as low as 7.0 mmol/L.

Box 1.2: Common symptoms of diabetes

Thirst
Polyuria/nocturia/incontinence in the elderly
Tiredness/lack of energy
Weight loss
Blurred vision
Genital irritation/thrush
Recurrent infections/boils
Mood changes
Tingling in hands and feet

Box 1.3: When should an OGTT be performed?

(1) If diabetes is suspected but there are no obvious symptoms and blood glucose values are equivocal
(2) During pregnancy
(3) When the diagnosis is in doubt or requires exclusion
(4) In epidemiological studies

The OGTT

The reliability of this test can be affected by the form of glucose ingested and the speed at which it is taken; attention to detail is therefore necessary (Keen and Barnes, 1997). Clear verbal and written information should be given to patients undergoing the test. The protocol in the laboratory should ensure that the glucose is consumed over 2–3 minutes.

> **Box 1.4: Patient instructions for a 75g OGTT**
>
> - Plenty of starchy food should be eaten for at least three days before the test. Starchy foods such as bread, potatoes, rice, pasta or cereals should be eaten at each meal. Three meals a day plus snacks should be eaten if possible
> - Fast overnight for 10–16 hours (only plain water can be taken)
> - Do not smoke for at least one hour before, and during, the test
> - Do not exercise during the test
> - Inform the lab of any illness such as sickness or diarrhoea and of any medication taken. The test may have to be postponed if you are unwell

The Classification of Diabetes

Once diagnosed, establishing the type of diabetes which an individual has may not always be clear cut.

MODY is not specifically mentioned in this classification. The discovery of genes implicated in MODY has increased interest in this condition.

Table 1.1: The diagnostic criteria for the diagnosis of diabetes and other categories of hyperglycaemia following a 75g OGTT

	Glucose concentration (mmol/L)		
	Venous whole blood	Capillary	Plasma venous
Diabetes Mellitus			
Fasting	≥ 6.1	≥ 6.1	≥ 7.0
2 hours after glucose load	≥ 10.0	≥ 11.1	≥ 11.1
Impaired glucose tolerance (IGT)			
Fasting (if measured)	< 6.1	< 6.1	< 7.0
2 hours after glucose load	≥ 6.7	≥ 7.8	≥ 7.8
Impaired fasting glycaemia (IFG)	≥ 5.6	≥ 5.6	≥ 6.1
Fasting	< 6.1	< 6.1	< 7.0
and (if measured) 2 hours after glucose load	< 6.7	< 7.8	< 7.8

Type 1 diabetes

A person with Type 1 diabetes is totally dependent on injected insulin to survive. If insulin replacement is not given, diabetic ketoacidosis will develop. Type 1 diabetes follows the autoimmune destruction of the β cells. High titres of islet cell antibodies in the blood of relatives of people with Type 1 diabetes impose an 80 per cent risk of developing Type 1 diabetes within 10 years. An inadequate C-peptide response to intravenous glucagon may help to differentiate Type 1 diabetes from Type 2 diabetes.

Box 1.5: WHO classification of diabetes and aetiological classification of disorders of glycaemia

Type 1 diabetes
Beta cell destruction usually leading to absolute insulin deficiency

Type 2 diabetes
May range from predominantly insulin resistance with relative insulin deficiency to a predominantly secretory defect with or without insulin resistance

Other specific types
Genetic defects of beta cell function
Genetic defects in insulin action
Diseases of the exocrine pancreas
Endocrinopathies
Drug or chemical induced
Infections
Uncommon forms of immune-mediated diabetes
Other genetic syndromes sometimes associated with diabetes

Gestational diabetes

Type 1 diabetes most commonly (but not exclusively) occurs in young people and children. There is a genetic link with the development of Type 1 diabetes; inheritance is polygenic. Those with HLA antigens DR3 and DR4 carry the greatest risk. Those with a father with Type 1 diabetes have a 6 per cent risk of developing it, a 3 per cent risk if the mother has diabetes and a 30 per cent risk if both parents have the disease. In studies using identical twins, if one twin has Type 1 diabetes there is only a 30–40 per cent chance that the other twin will develop it (Bowen Jones and Gill, 1997). Genetics is therefore only one risk factor.

Possible environmental triggers for Type 1 diabetes include a variety of viruses and neonatal exposure to bovine serum albumin in cows' milk.

The differential diagnosis of Type 1 diabetes is usually made on clinical judgement rather than C-peptide, islet cell antibodies and HLA testing, which may not be widely available.

Type 2 diabetes

Over 80 per cent of diabetes in Britain is Type 2 (Marks, 1996). Type 2 diabetes has traditionally been divided into two main groups: (a) obese; (b) non-obese. This distinction helps to distinguish between the underlying causes and helps to determine the most effective treatment.

Resistance to insulin plays a more important part in those who are overweight, whilst lack of insulin is more problematical in those who are thin or of normal body weight. Both mechanisms do, however, occur in both types to some degree.

The prevalence of Type 2 diabetes increases with age and it has a strong genetic link. The risks of a child developing Type 2 diabetes are about 15 per cent if one parent has the disease and 75 per cent if both are affected.

There is a 60–100 per cent chance of an identical twin of a patient with Type 2 diabetes developing the disease (Chiu and Permutt, 1997). Some races are more prone to Type 2 diabetes – for example, those from Southern Asia (see p. 161) – and may develop diabetes at an earlier age. The development of Type 2 diabetes also has strong environmental links. The risk of developing the disease increases with obesity and physical inactivity. There is a higher risk of Type 2 diabetes if the mother is affected (unlike Type 1 diabetes) and in those who were growth retarded due to poor intrauterine nutrition.

Different types of Type 2 diabetes have been discovered to have different modes of inheritance. For example, maturity-onset diabetes of the young (MODY) is heterogeneous genetically (see p. 10). Mitochondrial diabetes with deafness is inherited through the maternal line. Early-onset diabetes may occur in children born to two diabetic parents who receive a 'double dose' of Type 2 diabetes genes. Type 2 diabetes runs true to type; the individual is susceptible to the type of diabetes that other family members have.

Type 2 diabetes may present with symptoms of hyperglycaemia (see Box 1.2), with established long-term complications of diabetes, during an illness or on routine screening. Symptoms often occur over a long period and the patient is often over 30 years of age.

The Differential Diagnosis of Type 1 diabetes and Type 2 diabetes

There are a number of questions which are routinely asked of anyone referring a person with newly diagnosed diabetes by telephone to the diabetes centre in which I work. These help to determine whether the patient is likely to have Type 1 or Type 2 diabetes, and therefore the urgency of the appointment required (see Box 1.6).

> **Box 1.6: Questions asked if newly diagnosed**
>
> What is the result of the finger prick blood glucose?
> How old is the patient?
> Does the patient have symptoms of diabetes?
> - Are they thirsty?
> - How often do they get up to pass urine during the night?
> - Are they tired?
> - Do they feel ill?
> - Have they lost weight? If so, how much and over what period of time?
>
> How long has the patient had these symptoms?
> Has the patient got a family history of diabetes? If so, which type?
> Are there ketones in the urine? If so, how many, i.e. small/moderate/large, and when did the patient last eat?

The answers to these questions are interpreted as shown in Table 1.2.

Table 1.2: Differential diagnosis of Type 1 and Type 2 diabetes

Suspicion of Type 1 diabetes	Suspicion of Type 2 diabetes
Under 30 years of age	40 years of age and over
No family history of diabetes or family history of Type 1 diabetes	Family history of Type 2 diabetes
Severe symptoms of short duration	No symptoms or symptoms of long duration
Sudden and marked weight loss	No weight loss or small weight loss
Moderate/large amount of ketones in urine	No ketones or ketones associated with starvation
Presence of an autoimmune disease e.g. Graves' disease	No autoimmune disease

MODY

The more recent discovery, in the last six years, of the genes which cause MODY has led to increased interest in the condition. It also opens up the controversial area of the possibility of predictive genetic testing of family members of those with MODY.

According to Hattersley (1998) the definition of MODY should include early-onset Type 2 diabetes and autosomal dominant inheritance. Hattersley and Appleton (1997) define the diagnostic criteria for MODY as:

- early diagnosis of diabetes before the age of 25 years in at least one and usually two other family members

- Type 2 diabetes – confirmed by the absence of insulin treatment five years after diagnosis or, if treated with insulin, measurable C-peptide
- autosomal dominant inheritance (shown by vertical transmission of diabetes through at least three generations).

Each child of a parent with MODY has a 50 per cent risk of developing diabetes. Annual blood or urine tests for glucose are therefore recommended. MODY can result from different genes. Hattersley (1998) found that in 40 UK MODY pedigrees, 12 per cent had mutations in glucokinase, 65 per cent had mutations in hepatic nuclear factor 1 alpha (HNF1α), 5 per cent had mutations in hepatic nuclear factor 4 alpha (HNF4α) and 17.5 per cent were unexplained. The progression of diabetes and the treatment required differ according to the genes affected.

Patients with glucokinase mutations have a 'mild' form of diabetes. Hyperglycaemia is mild and begins in early childhood. Dietary restriction is usually all that is required except during pregnancy. Microvascular complications are rare. Those with mutations in the HNF1α gene are born with normoglycaemia and develop progressive hyperglycaemia due to severe and progressive beta cell dysfunction. Diabetes is usually diagnosed in adolescence or early adult life. Treatment involves diet in one-third of cases, tablets in one-third of cases and insulin in one-third of cases. A high incidence of microvascular complications is reported (Hattersley, 1998). Mutations in the HNF4α gene have a similar clinical history to that of HNF1α.

Impaired Glucose Tolerance (IGT)

The class IGT is now classified as a stage of impaired glucose regulation. It can be observed in any hyperglycaemic disorder and is not in itself diabetes. Of those with IGT, between 2 per cent and 5 per cent per year progress to Type 2 diabetes (Fitzgerald and Malins, 1976; Jarrett et al., 1979). The incidence of IGT increases with age and is associated with other risk factors for coronary heart disease. These include higher blood pressure, higher pulse rates and higher plasma triglyceride levels. IGT is a risk factor for cardiovascular disease. Those with IGT are not prone to the development of microvascular complications.

Impaired Fasting Glycaemia (IFG)

The category of IFG has been introduced by the WHO to classify individuals who have fasting glucose values above the normal range, but below those diagnostic of diabetes. IFG is not a clinical entity in its own right, but it is a risk factor for future diabetes.

National Service Framework

The NSF standards relevant to this chapter are shown in Box 1.7.

Box 1.7: NSF standards

Standard 1: Prevention of Type 2 diabetes
(1) The NHS will develop, implement and monitor strategies to reduce the risk of developing Type 2 diabetes in the population as a whole and to reduce the inequalities in the risk of developing Type 2 diabetes.

Standard 2: Identification of people with diabetes
(2) The NHS will develop, implement and monitor strategies to identify people who do not know they have diabetes.

The delivery strategy of the NSF recommends that Primary Care Trusts (PCTs) integrate their risk reduction strategies with local prevention programmes established under the NSF for CHD. The delivery strategy offers no suggestions for systematic screening for Type 2 diabetes. A pilot scheme will be undertaken.

Questions

(1) Simone's dad has Type 2 diabetes. She is concerned that she may develop diabetes too. What are the symptoms of hyperglycaemia that Simone should look out for? Why do these occur?

(2) Michael Abbott has 2 per cent glucose in his urine. Has he got diabetes? How can a diagnosis of diabetes be established?

(3) Sharon Richards has a blood glucose of 20.6 mmol/L when tested on the meter at the GP's surgery. Sharon asks you whether or not she is likely to have the type of diabetes that requires insulin. How would you determine whether she has Type 2 or Type 1 diabetes?

Suggested answers are found on pages 248–9.

References

Bowen Jones D, Gill GV (1997) Insulin dependent diabetes mellitus. In Pickup J, Williams G (Eds) Textbook of Diabetes 1997. 2nd edn. Oxford: Blackwell Science, 1, pp. 12.1–12.13.
Chiu KC, Permutt MA (1997) Genetic factors in the pathogenesis of non-insulin-dependent diabetes. In Pickup J, Williams G (Eds) Textbook of Diabetes 1997. 2nd edn. Oxford: Blackwell Science.

Department of Health (2001) National Service Framework for Diabetes – Standards: London.

Department of Health (2003) National Service Framework for Diabetes – Delivery Strategy: London.

The Expert Committee on the Diagnosis and Classification of Diabetes Mellitus (1997) Report of the Expert Committee on the Diagnosis and Classification of Diabetes Mellitus. Diabetes Care 20: 1183–97.

Fitzgerald MG, Malins JM (1976) Ten year follow up report on the Birmingham Diabetes Survey of 1961. BMJ ii: 35–7.

Hattersley AT (1998) Maturity-onset diabetes of the young: clinical heterogeneity explained by genetic heterogeneity. Diabetic Medicine 15: 15–24.

Hattersley A, Appleton M (1997) Two more diabetes genes identified. Diabetes Update Spring: 1–3.

Jarrett RJ, Keen H, Fuller JH, McCartney P (1979) Worsening of diabetes in men with impaired glucose tolerance. Diabetologia 16: 25–30.

Keen H, Barnes DJ (1997) The diagnosis and classification of diabetes mellitus and impaired glucose tolerance. In Pickup J, Williams G (Eds) Textbook of Diabetes 1997. 2nd edn. Oxford: Blackwell Science.

Marks L (1996) Counting the Cost – the Real Impact of Non-insulin Dependent Diabetes. London: Kings Fund/BDA.

World Health Organisation Expert Committee (1980) Second Report on Diabetes Mellitus. Technical Report Series 646. Geneva: WHO.

World Health Organisation Study Group (1985) Diabetes Mellitus. WHO Technical Report Series 727. Geneva: WHO.

World Health Organisation Department of Noncommunicable Disease Surveillance (1999) Report of a WHO Consultation. Definition, Diagnosis and Classification of Diabetes Mellitus and Its Complications. Part I Diagnosis and Classification of Diabetes Mellitus. Geneva: WHO.

Chapter 2
The treatment of diabetes

This chapter describes the types of treatment that are used in the management of Type 2 and Type 1 diabetes

Learning Outcomes

After reading this chapter you should be able to:

(1) provide clear accurate first-line dietary advice for those with both Type 2 and Type 1 diabetes
(2) suggest the drugs that would be most suitable for individuals with Type 2 diabetes
(3) demonstrate awareness of the benefits and disadvantages of at least two different types of insulin regimes.

The main aims of treatment are:

- to relieve the symptoms of hyperglycaemia (polydipsia, polyuria, etc.) and to prevent the development of ketosis in those with Type 1 diabetes
- to minimize the risks of hypoglycaemia (a side-effect of sulphonylurea drugs and insulin injections)
- to prevent or minimize the long-term macrovascular and microvascular complications of diabetes.

Type 2 diabetes can be treated using dietary modification alone, dietary modification and oral hypoglycaemic drugs, or dietary modification and insulin. Those with Type 1 diabetes require insulin injections; they produce no insulin of their own and are therefore dependent on insulin injections for survival. If insulin treatment is required in a patient with Type 2 diabetes the diabetes may be described as insulin-treated diabetes (ITD). These individuals are not dependent on insulin.

Diet

Dietary modification is important in the treatment of diabetes. Lean et al. (1992) claim that dietary advice for those with Type 1 diabetes and those with Type 2 diabetes is essentially the same and should mirror the advice given to the population as a whole. Although cardiovascular diseases are the major cause of mortality for both types of diabetes, Lean et al. (1992) argue that restriction of saturated fats should be given greater emphasis in Type 2 diabetes where lipid abnormalities are more common and clearly related to cardiovascular disease. Protein restriction which attempts to modify the progression of microvascular disease should be directed more towards those with Type 1 diabetes. They also state that it is important to adopt a dietary policy that is clear and consistent for both types of diabetes and that this will ensure credibility with patients and the general public.

Dietary recommendations should be based on the current eating habits and lifestyle of the individual. Factors such as age, financial status, occupation, body weight, presence of hyperlipidaemia, hypertension and other medical conditions need to be considered. It is important that every patient with diabetes be seen by a state-registered dietitian and have an individual diet prescription. Other health care professionals need to understand the basic principles of the 'diabetic diet' to provide 'first aid' dietary advice before the patient is seen by a dietitian.

Specific dietary considerations for those from ethnic minority groups, the elderly and those planning a pregnancy are discussed in Chapter 6; how to manage carbohydrate replacement when ill is discussed in Chapter 5.

Dietary Recommendations for those with Diabetes (based on the British Diabetic Association (BDA) Report, 1992) (Note: BDA has been Diabetes UK since 2000)

Regular food intake

This is particularly important for those treated with sulphonylureas or insulin as they are prone to hypoglycaemia if meals are delayed or missed. Three well-spaced meals are usually adequate for those taking oral hypoglycaemic agents but snacks between meals are usually needed for those treated with insulin. Splitting daily food intake has been shown to increase insulin sensitivity (Jenkins et al., 1989). Snacks may be less necessary if a basal bolus insulin regime (clear insulin before each meal and cloudy insulin before bed) is used, particularly if the type of clear insulin used is lispro (Gale, 1996) or aspart.

Energy intake

The amount of calories required by each individual should be assessed by the dietitian. Tables are used to predict individual energy requirements based on sex, body weight and energy expended by physical exercise. In addition, a dietary history should be taken.

Acceptable body weight is one which corresponds to a body mass index (BMI) of between 20 and 25 kg/m². In order to calculate BMI the patient's weight and height should be measured and the formula shown below used.

$$BMI = \frac{\text{Weight in kilograms}}{(\text{height in metres})^2}$$

The waist–hip ratio can be used as an indicator of obesity in addition to BMI. Coronary heart disease is linked with central obesity (apple rather than pear shaped). Being apple shaped is more common in some ethnic groups. A waist–hip ratio of less than 1.0 in men or 0.8 in women is desirable.

Weight-reducing diets should generally aim for an energy deficit of 500 Kcal/day, which leads to a weight loss of around 0.5 kg per week. It is important that weight loss does not exceed 2 kg/week as greater weight loss would suggest a breakdown of muscle rather than fat (Ha and Lean, 1997). A target weight loss should be agreed with the patient.

Weight loss reduces cardiovascular risk factors. It lowers blood pressure, decreases triglyceride levels and very-low-density lipoprotein (VLDL) concentrations and increases high-density lipoprotein (HDL) concentrations. In addition, weight loss in those with Type 2 diabetes improves insulin secretion, enhances insulin sensitivity and decreases blood glucose.

Carbohydrate (starch)

At least 50 per cent of calorie intake should come from carbohydrate-containing foods. This figure is similar to the amount of carbohydrate eaten by the general population (45 per cent). However, the general population in the UK obtain 10–20 per cent of their dietary energy from sugars, mainly sucrose. For those with diabetes it is recommended that the intake of sucrose be reduced.

In the past people with diabetes were advised to restrict carbohydrate-containing foods. It is therefore difficult for some to believe that a high carbohydrate diet is good for them. For example, many still believe that bananas are too high in sugar and should therefore be avoided.

Different types of carbohydrate foods have been shown to have different glycaemic responses. This 'glycaemic index' has been proposed as a basis for a diabetic diet. Food such as pasta, porridge, beans, peas and lentils, as well as

'Rich Tea' biscuits and biscuits containing oats, and fruit (fresh, dried or tinned) have been shown to have a low glycaemic index and may offer benefits in terms of lipid reduction. Gordon (1996) claims that most glycaemic index studies have been carried out on single foods; the effect of a food taken as part of a mixed meal is therefore unknown. Lean et al. (1992) claim that the glycaemic index is too complicated to be used directly with patients, although they recommend that 'slow release' low glycaemic index foods form a major component of each meal.

However, others have argued that low glycaemic index foods have been shown to improve overall blood glucose control in Type 2 diabetes (Wolever, 1997; Frost et al., 1994). Low glycaemic foods are absorbed more slowly, which may be particularly beneficial for preventing nocturnal hypoglycaemia (Frost et al., 1994).

Box 2.1: The two types of carbohydrate

(1) Monosaccharides or refined carbohydrates or simple sugars:
  e.g. sugary drinks, honey, sweets, chocolate
(2) Polysaccharides or complex carbohydrates:
  e.g. bread, potatoes, pasta, rice, fruit

Foods such as sweets and chocolates are rapidly absorbed into the bloodstream elevating blood glucose levels in those with diabetes. These foods should be reserved for treats or special occasions and ideally be eaten after a fibre-containing meal which will help to delay absorption. Sweets and chocolate may be necessary to prevent hypoglycaemia during exercise (see p. 146). Sugary drinks such as colas, Lucozade or tea containing sugar should be avoided and used only in emergencies to treat hypoglycaemia or to manage illness if the patient is unable to eat normally.

Complex carbohydrates take longer to be broken down into glucose and lead to a more gradual rise in blood glucose levels.

Sugar

The diet recommended for those with diabetes is 'low sugar' rather than 'no sugar'. Up to 25g (1 oz) per day of sucrose can be consumed as part of an overall diet that is low in fats and high in fibre. Foods which are obviously sweet such as sweets, chocolates, iced cakes, etc. need to be restricted, rather than products which may contain a little sugar. In practical terms the amount of sugar in tinned baked beans or soup is negligible when taken as part of a healthy diet.

When people are first diagnosed with diabetes they may feel that they need to (or may have been told to) avoid sugar altogether and may stop eating high-fibre breakfast cereals or even bread, which both contain some sugar. Providing that sugar is not the main ingredient these foods will not affect blood glucose control.

Sugar may be required to give bulk in some recipes, particularly in cakes. Many recipes can be successfully adapted using half the usual quantity of sugar. Diabetes UK produce a booklet entitled *Home Baking* which includes practical tips for home baking and recipes containing less sugar and less fat.

Artificial sweeteners rather than sugar should be used in drinks, custards and on cereals; these have no effect on blood glucose levels.

Those with Type 1 diabetes will need some understanding of the carbohydrate content of foods so that similar amounts can be taken on a daily basis and to enable accurate adjustment of insulin doses if the amount of carbohydrate is increased or decreased. Some patients may use carbohydrate exchange lists. These exchange systems are based on patients being taught the carbohydrate values of various foods and how to exchange them for others with similar carbohydrate values. For example, a digestive biscuit may be swapped for an apple as both supply approximately 10 g of carbohydrate. Lean et al. (1992) argue that the blood glucose response to food is influenced by many factors in addition to the amount of carbohydrate that it contains. These factors include the content of fat, dietary fibre, the physical form of food (the shape of pasta makes a difference), water content, temperature and how much the food is chewed. Exchange lists may therefore be misleading. Carbohydrate counting is used most commonly when a continuous subcutaneous insulin infusion (CSII) pump is used and on the DAFNE education programme (please see p. 108).

Carbohydrate exchange systems have advantages and disadvantages. Many patients treated with insulin may have used them for some years. It is therefore important for nurses to have some idea of how they work. Carbohydrate exchange systems may give confidence to newly diagnosed patients. Many such patients like to know 'exactly' how much they can have but gradually learn to gauge amounts and swap carbohydrate-containing foods without actually needing to count the carbohydrates each time. Exchange systems may also be helpful to professionals advising on insulin adjustment. It is very useful to have some idea of how much carbohydrate the dietitian has recommended that the patient should eat and its distribution throughout the day. The patient may need to eat more food rather than reduce the insulin dose to prevent hypoglycaemia, if eating less than advised by the dietitian.

It is useful for insulin-treated patients to be familiar with carbohydrate exchanges in order to deal with intercurrent illness. Diabetes UK, (see BDA, 1996–7b) recommend replacing the usual amount of carbohydrate with sugary drinks if the patient is unable to eat solid food. This is very difficult to do if the patient is unaware how much carbohydrate he or she usually eats.

A disadvantage of the carbohydrate exchange system is that it does not take into account the fat, energy or protein content or glycaemic index of foods. A digestive biscuit may be equivalent in terms of carbohydrate to an apple (see Table 2.1) but it contains more fat and more calories and may therefore not be an ideal swap for someone who is trying to lose weight. Carbohydrate exchange systems have also been used in the past to restrict carbohydrate intake and may encourage increased fat intake. Liquid forms of carbohydrate are more quickly absorbed than foods high in fibre, and do not sustain blood glucose levels for as long. Lucozade would therefore not be suitable to swap with bread or biscuits for a before-bed snack.

The ability to multiply and divide is necessary in order for patients to use carbohydrate exchange lists successfully. This may be difficult for some patients and may discourage a varied diet.

Table 2.1: Carbohydrate (CHO) exchange list

Food	Amount necessary to give 10g CHO	Calorie content	Fat content
Wholemeal/ white bread	1 slice	47 Kcals	0.38 g
Digestive biscuit	1 biscuit	68 Kcals	3.0 g
Banana	½ banana	41 Kcals	0.1 g
Apple	1 apple	40 Kcals	0.09 g
Crisps	1 bag	110 Kcals	7.6 g
Lucozade	50 ml	36 Kcals	0 g

Some centres in the UK and in Europe no longer use formal carbohydrate exchange lists, preferring meal plans or the 'plate model' which was originally advocated by the Swedish Diabetic Association (1987). This has been adapted by the Health Education Authority (1996).

The plate is divided into three sections. The smallest section (approximately one-fifth of the total) is for meat, fish, eggs or cheese and the remaining area is divided into two roughly equal proportions. One is for rice, potatoes, pasta, bread, etc. and the other for vegetables or fruit. Patients are given ideas for 'swaps' but grams of carbohydrate are not mentioned and carbohydrate is referred to in the overall context of a 'healthy' balanced diet.

Fibre

Fibre consists of non-starch polysaccharides, which are a type of carbohydrate. A fibre intake of 30 g per day is recommended for those with diabetes, again similar to that for the general population. There are two types of fibre; soluble and insoluble. Insoluble fibre is found in foods such as wholemeal bread, flour, pasta, brown rice and high-fibre breakfast cereal. Peas, beans, lentils, oats and fruit are good sources of soluble fibre. Insoluble fibre can help patients to feel full and may assist weight loss (Garrow and Owens, 1990). Soluble fibre is felt to be most effective in improving blood glucose, HbA1$_c$ and serum total and LDL-cholesterol concentrations (Fuessl et al., 1987). Pulses such as peas, sweetcorn, beans, lentils, oats and fruit should therefore be encouraged.

Box 2.2: Tips to increase fibre intake

- Add baked beans/kidney beans/sweetcorn to pasta sauces or mince (they are a cheap way to add 'bulk' too)
- Choose fruit for snacks – aim for 3–4 pieces per day
- Eat plenty of vegetables
- Eat boiled potatoes in the skins or jacket potatoes
- Choose rye, wholegrain, wholewheat, granary or high-fibre white bread (if white bread is preferred or patients are on a tight budget, white bread is much cheaper; add baked beans to make a high fibre meal or have fruit with a sandwich)
- Eat wholegrain breakfast cereals or porridge
- Try wholemeal pasta/brown rice
- If biscuits or crackers are eaten choose the wholegrain varieties (please note these can be high in fat)

Fat

People with diabetes have a high risk of ischaemic vascular disease and it is therefore recommended that fat should make up less than 35 per cent of total energy requirements. The Nutrition Study Group of the European Association for the Study of Diabetes (1988) recommended that energy derived from fat should be about 30 per cent of total energy but found that higher intakes of fat, mostly from olive oil, occur in Mediterranean countries and are associated with lower risks of heart disease. The main aim therefore is to reduce the intake of saturated fat. Diabetes UK (formerly the BDA) recommend 10 per cent saturated fats, 10 per cent polyunsaturated fats and 10–15 per cent monounsaturated fats.

Lean et al. (1992) claim that for those with diabetes fat reduction is the most difficult dietary recommendation to follow.

Box 2.3: Sources of fat

(1) Saturated fats:
   e.g. red meat, fat on meat, lard, dripping, butter, full-fat cheese
(2) Polyunsaturated fats:
   e.g. sunflower oil, safflower oil, corn oil, soya oil and ranges of spreads and margarines based on these products; oily fish, e.g. pilchards (these also contain omega 3 fatty acids and can protect against heart disease)
(3) Monounsaturated fats:
   e.g. olive oil, rapeseed oil and products such as spreads based on these

---

Foods which contain cholesterol, such as eggs, tend to have little effect on blood cholesterol levels; the principal dietary influence on serum cholesterol levels is the intake of saturated fats. Stringent restriction of dietary cholesterol is therefore not recommended.

Box 2.4: Tips to reduce fat intake

- Use skimmed or semi-skimmed rather than full fat milk
- Choose a low-fat spread high in mono- or polyunsaturates and spread thinly
- Grill, boil, bake, microwave, steam or poach rather than fry
- Eat less meat and choose chicken (without the skin) and fish more often
- Use more pulses and vegetables in pasta sauces, cottage pie, etc. and therefore less meat
- Measure oil rather than pouring directly from the pot; gradually reduce the amount
- Use ghee sparingly
- Choose lean meat and trim off the fat
- Try to eat fewer pies and sausages
- Reduce the amount of biscuits and cakes; have fruit instead
- Have less cheese. Use stronger flavoured cheese and slice thinly or grate or try low-fat cheeses such as Edam.
- Try using low-fat yogurt or fromage frais rather than double cream

---

Reducing fat intake will reduce energy (calorie) intake and therefore lead to weight loss. Fat contains over twice as many calories per gram as either carbohydrate or protein.

Patients of normal body weight already consume the right amount of energy for them. It is therefore important if fat intake is decreased that calorie intake is increased from complex carbohydrates to prevent undesirable weight loss.

Protein

Limitation of protein intake is more likely to be necessary in those with Type 1 diabetes as nephropathy is more common than in those with Type 2 diabetes. There is some evidence (Zeller et al., 1991) that protein restriction slows progressive renal failure in those with Type 1 diabetes. Diabetes UK recommend that about 12 per cent of total energy intake be obtained from protein for those with early nephropathy. They claim that evidence supporting protein restriction for all with diabetes is weak, and recommend that other groups with diabetes should avoid a higher than average protein intake.

Salt

Hypertension is common in those with Type 2 diabetes and can be reduced through weight loss and sodium restriction. Salt may be hidden in foods; products such as ready-made meals, tinned foods and some take-aways may be high in salt.

Box 2.5: Tips to reduce salt intake

- Use fewer packaged or processed foods. If tinned vegetables are used choose those with no added salt
- Use less salt in cooking; use herbs and spices for flavour instead
- Taste food before adding salt at the table – you might not need it!
- Eat fewer salty foods such as smoked fish, bacon, crisps
- Gradually reduce the amount of salt to become accustomed to the taste change

---

Alcohol

The weekly 'limits' are the same as those recommended by the Health Education Authority for the general population. These are 21 units for men and 14 units for women

---

Box 2.6: How much is one unit of alcohol?

Beer/lager/cider – ½ pint
Sherry/vermouth/liqueur/aperitif – 1 pub measure
Wine – 1 standard wine glass
Spirits – 1 pub measure

Alcohol inhibits gluconeogenesis (glucose production by the liver). There is therefore a risk of hypoglycaemia occurring if alcohol is drunk by those treated with sulphonylureas or insulin. This can occur several hours after the alcohol is taken. Low carbohydrate drinks which are high in alcohol should therefore be avoided. Alcohol should never be taken on an empty stomach and should ideally be drunk with a meal which is high in carbohydrate. Patients should be advised not to save up their units and binge. If patients are likely to binge, e.g. at Christmas or on special occasions, extra high-fibre carbohydrate snacks should be taken, particularly before bed. Patients should also be warned that the symptoms of 'hypos' may go unrecognized by themselves or others if they have been drinking. Some form of identification should be worn and friends warned about the possibility of hypoglycaemia.

Drinks with a high carbohydrate content such as sweet sherries, sweet wines and sweet liqueurs should also be avoided. Patients who are overweight should be advised to limit their alcohol intake to one unit per day as alcohol is high in calories. For example, half a pint of beer or lager contains 90 Kcal, a glass of dry white wine 70 Kcal and a pub measure of spirit 65 Kcal.

Fruit and vegetables

Five portions of fruit and vegetables should be eaten per day to reduce the risk of heart disease (Department of Health, 1994). Fruit can be used for snacks, salad (pre-washed for the non-domesticated) can be added to pizza or ready-made meals and sweetcorn/kidney beans to stews and sauces. Examples of a portion include:

- 1 small banana, 1 apple or 1 orange
- 2 clementines
- 1/2 a mango
- handful of grapes
- 3 tablespoons of stewed/tinned fruit in juice
- 2 heaped tablespoons of any vegetable

Diabetic foods

Thomas et al. (1992) claim that diabetic foods offer no physiological or psychological benefits and have no place in the modern management of diabetes. 'Diabetic' foods are expensive, costing between one and a half and four times as much as their ordinary equivalents. There is a huge variety of reduced sugar/low-calorie products such as reduced-sugar jams, sugar-free jellies, etc. These products are cheaper and are often lower in fat and calories than 'diabetic' foods. Diabetic foods may contain sorbitol and fructose, which can cause diarrhoea. The availability of diabetic products appears to undermine the philosophy that the diabetic diet is healthy eating, suitable for everybody. Many patients may feel that diabetic products are superior and necessary because they are sold by chemists. Nurses should strongly advise patients not to buy these products. If chocolate or sweets are desired, small amounts of ordinary chocolate or sweets should be taken after a meal high in complex carbohydrate.

Summary

- Diet should be based on individual requirements, taking account of weight, occupation, financial status, ethnic group, etc.
- All patients should be seen by a dietitian.
- Ideally BMI should be between 20 and 25.
- Regular meals should be taken.
- Obvious sugar and sugar in drinks should be replaced with sweeteners (sugar in savoury products or as part of wholegrain breakfast cereals is fine).
- High-fibre carbohydrate foods should form the main part of each meal.
- Total fat intake should be reduced and saturated fats substituted for polyunsaturated and monounsaturated fats.
- Three or four pieces of fruit should be eaten each day.
- Plenty of vegetables and salad should be eaten.
- Salt should be reduced.
- Alcohol should be limited.
- Diabetic products should be avoided.

Common Dietary Misconceptions

- Food should be withheld if the blood glucose is high, in order to lower blood glucose. This is done particularly at bedtime. Meals and snacks should be taken irrespective of blood glucose levels. The before-bed snack is taken to prevent nocturnal hypoglycaemia. Withholding this snack is likely to lead to hypoglycaemia even if the blood glucose before bed is high. Tablets and insulin should be adjusted to complement a healthy diet.
- People with diabetes should reduce 'starchy' foods such as bread and potatoes. Bananas have been given a particularly bad press. Most people need to eat more of these foods.
- Honey and brown sugar are healthy and do not elevate blood glucose levels. They are in fact refined carbohydrates like white sugar.
- Unsweetened orange juice is low in sugar and can be drunk freely. This is untrue, it contains similar amounts of sugar to ordinary lemonade.
- Low-fat foods are also low in sugar. This is not necessarily true; low-fat Horlicks contains more sugar and more calories than ordinary instant drinking chocolate.
- Low-fat digestive biscuits and crisps are low in fat and help weight loss. Low-fat biscuits and crisps still contain more calories than fruit.

As a nurse, it may be necessary for you to give the first-line dietary advice to a newly diagnosed patient or to try to establish reasons for a patient's poor blood glucose control. Perhaps the following two case-studies may give you some food for thought.

Case-study 2.1

John Smith is 50 years of age and has been recently diagnosed as having Type 2 diabetes. He takes no medication, his BMI is 30 and he looks rather plump. His capillary blood glucose is 18 mmol/L and he complains of thirst, tiredness and having to get up at least four times during the night to pass urine.

What questions might you ask Mr Smith with regard to his diet and lifestyle?

- Does he have sugar in drinks? How much? How many sugary drinks does he have a day? Ask specifically about tea/coffee, fizzy drinks and fresh fruit juice.
- Does he eat regularly? How many meals does he have a day?
- What does he usually eat? Does he have snacks – if so, what? Any puddings or desserts?
- Does he do any exercise, such as walking, gardening, etc?

Mr Smith answered in the following way:

- He takes 3 teaspoons of sugar in his tea and coffee and drinks approximately 10 cups of tea a day. Since he has been thirsty he has also taken between 3 and 6 litres of ordinary fizzy drinks a day in addition to 2 pints of full-fat milk.
- He regularly eats two meals a day. The first is breakfast in the transport café, consisting of a fried egg, two rashers of bacon, a sausage, baked beans and two slices of toast. He meets other drivers for breakfast, which is a valuable social activity. Breakfasts at the weekend are similar.

  A chocolate bar or packet of crisps is eaten for lunch.

  The evening meal is cooked by Mrs Smith and usually consists of either meat, potatoes and vegetables, spaghetti bolognese, pie and chips, a roast, or sausage, mash and beans. He doesn't usually have dessert, except on Sundays when he has apple pie and custard.
- He works as a driver and does little exercise; Mrs Smith does the gardening and walks the dog whilst he is at work.

What first-line dietary advice would you give?

- Explain why a change in diet will be necessary, i.e. for the relief of symptoms and the risk reduction of cardiovascular disease.
- Stop sugar in tea and coffee and try sweeteners instead. Try diet drinks or water to quench thirst rather than sugary drinks and milk.
- Change from full-fat milk to semi-skimmed and try to reduce to one pint per day.
- Try to eat three meals a day; perhaps have a sandwich or a roll rather than chocolate or crisps for lunch.
- Reduce the amount of fried food. Perhaps have cereal and toast at the weekends and try beans on toast a couple of times during the week.
- Try to make potatoes or bread the largest part of each meal, and meat the smallest.
- Perhaps try to take the dog for a walk in the evening.

This is a lot of information to take in at one time. It may need to be introduced more slowly and will almost certainly need to be reviewed. It is most likely that stopping sugar in drinks alone, even if no other advice is followed, would lead to a dramatic improvement in symptoms and blood glucose levels. Dietary measures may be sufficient to control Mr Smith's diabetes.

Case-study 2.2

Karen Beale is 30 years old and has had diabetes for 10 years. She takes insulin twice a day and has unstable diabetes. Her home blood glucose measurements range between 2 and 19 mmol/L and she has at least five hypos a week. She is terrified of gaining weight, her BMI is 26 and she often misses meals and snacks.

How would you advise Karen before her dietitian's appointment next week?

- Reassure Karen that you do not wish her to gain weight either.
- Assess what Karen eats. Look at fat content in addition to carbohydrate-containing foods. Can the fat content and therefore the calorie intake be reduced? If crisps, biscuits, cheese, fried food or take-aways are eaten, perhaps try to exchange these for fruit, bread, pasta or rice, which contain fewer calories and may prevent hypoglycaemia.
- Explain the importance of preventing hypoglycaemia. Hypos necessitate treatment with sugar, they make patients hungry and are often treated or followed with high-calorie foods such as biscuits or chocolate. Preventing hypoglycaemia with regular low-fat high-fibre carbohydrate meals and snacks will reduce calories.
- Advise Karen to eat three meals a day, the largest part of which should be carbohydrate, and snacks of fruit or a slice of bread mid-morning, mid-afternoon and before bed.

Treatment of Type 2 diabetes

Oral hypoglycaemic agents should not be introduced until diet has been tried for three months in those with Type 2 diabetes, according to Fox and Pickering (1995a). They do, however, accept that if after a month on a diet the patient remains symptomatic with a fasting blood glucose greater than 12 mmol/L, starting tablets is justified. There is a danger of hypoglycaemia if sulphonlyureas are started too quickly in patients whose blood glucose may still be falling due to the effects of changes to the diet. If a patient's diet has been assessed and found to be healthy at diagnosis, with few or no changes required, tablets may be necessary from the outset.

Few patients with Type 2 diabetes respond to dietary modification alone (Ha and Lean, 1997). The United Kingdom Prospective Diabetes Study (UKPDS, 1995) found that diet alone maintained fasting plasma glucose at less than 6 mmol/L for three years in only 3–4 per cent of those with Type 2 diabetes. Most overweight patients with Type 2 diabetes will fail to achieve sufficient weight loss to control blood glucose and lipid levels with diet and lifestyle advice (e.g. exercise) alone after 3–6 months. Diabetes UK (see BDA, 1996–7a) estimate that 50 per cent of those with Type 2 diabetes are treated with tablets, 20 per cent with diet alone and 30 per cent with insulin.

Whichever method is chosen to treat diabetes it is important that diet, particularly fat reduction, a reduction in total energy intake (in those who are overweight) and increased physical exercise are used in conjunction with the regime (Groop, 1997).

There are currently six groups of oral agents used to treat Type 2 diabetes: (1) sulphonylureas; (2) biguanides; (3) alpha-glucosidase inhibitors; (4) thiazolidinediones; (5) meglitinides (e.g. Repaglinide); (6) amino acid derivatives (e.g. Nateglinide). The most important decision is which is most suitable for the individual patient. The actions of these drugs and their potential side-effects will be discussed and case-studies used to illustrate how they can be used.

Sulphonylureas

Action

Sulphonylureas stimulate the release of insulin by pancreatic beta cells, reduce hepatic glucose production and increase insulin-mediated uptake of glucose in peripheral tissues (Chan and MacFarlane, 1988). The main difference in practice between sulphonylureas is the duration of action. Chlorpropamide and glibenclamide have a long half-life, chlorpropamide 24–48 hours and glibenclamide 10–20 hours (Fox and Pickering, 1995a). This can lead to long-lasting severe hypoglycaemia and even death. These drugs should not be used to treat the elderly or those in renal failure as they are excreted by the kidneys. Elderly patients are best treated with shorter-acting drugs such as tolbutamide or gliclazide which are inactivated and excreted by the liver (Chan and MacFarlane, 1988).

Side-effects

Other than hypoglycaemia, reported side-effects of sulphonylureas are rare. They may occasionally cause skin rashes, gastrointestinal symptoms, headache or blood dyscrasias. Chlorpropamide (rarely used in modern diabetes management) causes facial flushing after alcohol ingestion and may lead to water retention and hyponatraemia.

Many patients report hunger and weight gain. Fox and Pickering (1995a) attribute this to improved blood glucose control with less glucose (and therefore fewer calories) lost in the urine and to a sense of well-being which may lead to an increase in appetite. Another possible cause of weight gain could be over-treatment; patients overeat to prevent hypoglycaemia. Grant and Marsden (1991b) argue that sulphonlyureas should be avoided in those who are obese as they cause insulin hypersecretion (insulin is anabolic) and weight gain.

Timing

Sulphonylureas should be taken 30 minutes before a meal as this has been shown to result in lower post-prandial plasma blood glucose levels than when taken with the meal (Melander et al., 1989).

Doses

It is usual to increase the dosage gradually to the maximum recommended level if treatment goals are not achieved on lower doses. Groop (1997) argues that sulphonlyureas operate within a narrow range of plasma concentrations which

can be achieved with relatively low doses. Grant and Marsden (1991b) argue
that they either work, or do not, quickly.

Table 2.2: Some commonly used sulphonylureas

Drug	Tablet size	Dose	Duration of effect (Groop, 1997)
Gliclazide (Diamicron)	80 mg	40–320 mg daily Up to 160 mg as a single dose. Higher doses divided into twice a day	10–15 hours
Glibenclamide (Daonil, Euglucon)	2.5mg or 5mg	2.5–15 mg once a day.	20–24 hours
Glipizide (Glibenese, Minodiab)	2.5 mg or 5 mg	2.5mg – 40mg daily. 15 mg as a single dose. Higher doses divided, twice or three times a day.	12–14 hours
Tolbutamide (Rastinon, Glyconon, Pramidex)	500 mg	500–2000 mg daily. Usually given in divided doses three times a day.	6–10 hours
Chlorpropamide (Diabinese, Glymese)	100 mg or 250 mg	100mg- 500mg once a day.	24–72 hours
Tolazamide (Tolanase)	100 mg or 250 mg	100–1000 mg daily. Usually divided into a three times a day regime.	16–24 hours
Glimepiride (Amaryl)	1 mg, 2 mg, 3 mg, or 4 mg	1–4 mg daily (exceptionally 6 mg may be used).	24 hours (serum half-life 5–8 hours) (Hoechst, 2001)

The cost of the different sulphonylurea drugs, in addition to the duration of
action and method of excretion, may also influence which drugs are most
commonly prescribed (Grant and Marsden, 1991b). Drugs such as
chlorpropamide, tolbutamide and glibenclamide are significantly cheaper to
prescribe at an average dose than gliclazide, glipizide or tolazamide.

Box 2.7: Use of sulphonylureas

- Sulphonylureas should be used in patients of normal or below normal body weight, after dietary modification has failed
- Tablets should be taken before food (ideally 30 minutes before)
- Chlorpropamide and glibenclamide should not be used in the elderly or those with renal impairment

---

Biguanides

Metformin is the only available biguanide in Britain. Groop (1997) claims that metformin should be considered as an anti-hyperglycaemic rather than a hypoglycaemic agent as it does not lower blood glucose concentrations below normal levels.

Action

No single explanation has been found to account for the anti-hyperglycaemic action of metformin; it is considered to have small effects on multiple meta-bolic pathways (Groop, 1997). Stumvoll et al. (1995) argue that its main metabolic effects on those with Type 2 diabetes are to inhibit gluconeogenesis and decrease hepatic glucose output. Chan and MacFarlane (1988) cite the main effects of metformin as increased peripheral uptake of glucose and delayed gastrointestinal absorption of glucose, in addition to inhibition of gluconeogenesis.

Metformin has been associated with weight loss (Clarke and Campbell, 1977, Chan and MacFarlane, 1988) and has been shown to reduce elevated lipid concentrations (Wu et al., 1990).

Unlike sulphonylurea therapy, metformin is not associated with weight gain. Metformin is therefore most suitable for overweight persons with Type 2 diabetes.

Side-effects

The most serious is the risk of lactic acidosis but this is very rare and can largely be avoided by not using metformin in high-risk patients. There is higher risk of lactic acidosis in those with renal, hepatic or cardiac failure and when there is tissue anoxia or in the presence of alcohol (Fox and Pickering, 1995a).

Gastrointestinal side-effects are relatively common with metformin. These can be minimized by educating patients to take metformin immediately after meals and by gradually increasing the dose. A metallic taste, which is due to excretion of metformin by the salivary glands, and decreased vitamin B12 absorption may also occur.

Dose

The usual starting dose is 500 mg once or twice a day gradually increasing to a maximum of 3 g in 24 hours, although in practice most clinicians limit the dose to 2 g a day. Both 500 mg and 850 mg tablets are produced. Common regimes are 850 mg twice daily, 500 mg three times a day or 1 g daily after meals. Metformin may be combined with sulphonylureas, and alpha-glucosidase inhibitors, thiazolidinediones, repaglinide, nateglinide or insulin.

Alpha-glucosidase inhibitors

Acarbose (Glucobay) is the only alpha-glucosidase inhibitor available in Britain.

Action

Acarbose delays and reduces carbohydrate absorption in the small intestine and reduces post-prandial glucose peaks. It is most effective in patients with a high carbohydrate intake.

Side-effects

These nearly all affect the gastrointestinal tract. The main side-effect is flatulence with abdominal distension and pain. Diarrhoea may also occur. For this reason acarbose is contraindicated in those with inflammatory bowel disease (e.g. ulcerative colitis), predisposition to intestinal obstruction, large hernias and a history of abdominal surgery. It is also contraindicated in hepatic and severe renal impairment. 'Wind' can be extremely embarrassing in particular to middle-aged and elderly women. Acarbose should be introduced slowly to minimize these effects.

Dose and timing

Initially 50 mg once a day, chewed with the first mouthful of the main meal. This should be continued for two weeks and then if there are no gastrointestinal symptoms the dose can be increased to twice a day for two weeks and then three times a day (see Figure 2.1).

Acarbose may be increased to 100 mg three times daily after 6–8 weeks. The maximum dose is 200 mg three times a day, but patients on this dose need to have serum transaminase levels checked once a month for a period of six months.

If used in conjunction with a sulphonylurea, hypoglycaemia is possible. Hypoglycaemia should be treated with glucose *not* sucrose as acarbose inhibits the metabolism and subsequent absorption of sucrose.

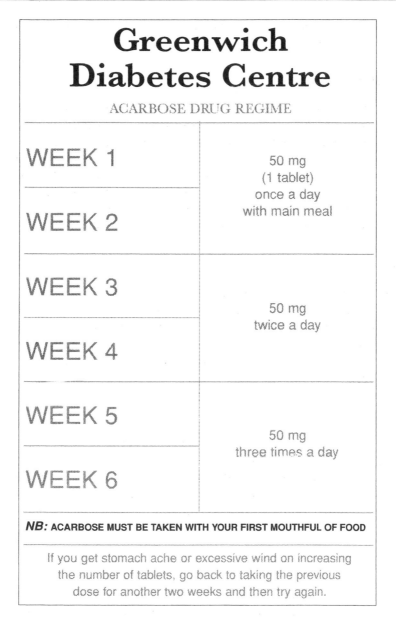

Figure 2.1: Acarbose patient advice leaflet

Use

Acarbose, like metformin, does not lead to weight gain. It is therefore most suitable for those who are overweight and for whom diet therapy alone has failed. It is recommended that acarbose be used as a first-line therapy before the introduction of sulphonylureas or metformin. However the unpleasant side-effects and the familiarity of clinicians with the other drugs means that it may still be used as a last resort.

Thiazolidinediones

Troglitazone (Romozin) was introduced in October 1997 as the only thiazolidinedione available in Britain for the treatment of Type 2 diabetes. The drug was, however, suspended in the UK on 29 November 1997 after reports of severe hepatic dysfunction. Since that time rosiglitazone and pioglitazone have been endorsed by the National Institute for Clinical Excellence (NICE) (August 2000; March 2001). Glitazones are licensed for use with either sulphonylureas or metformin (not both together) in patients who fail to achieve adequate glucose control despite maximum tolerated doses of oral monotherapy.

Action

The main function of glitazones is to reduce insulin and thus improve glucose uptake, although they have also been shown to improve pancreatic beta cell function. Glitazones are contraindicated in liver disease or if transaminases are more than 2.5 times normal levels. They are also contraindicated in congestive cardiac failure, severe renal impairment and pregnancy.

Side-effects

These include anaemia, headache, dizziness, gastrointestinal disturbances and weight gain (0.7–2.3 kg). Rosiglitazone has been shown to cause small increases in cholesterol, LDL and triglycerides but also in favourable HDL. Pioglitazone has been shown to significantly reduce triglyceride concentrations with no significant increase in LDL. Hypoglycaemia has also been reported.

Dose

For rosiglitazone the starting dose is 4 mg daily, which should be reassessed at 8 weeks. The maximum dose is 8 mg. rosiglitazone should be given once a day and can be taken with or without food. For pioglitazone the dose is 30 mg once a day, irrespective of meal times.

Use

The use of rosiglitazone and pioglitazone has been approved by NICE (2000; 2001) as an add-on therapy. They can be used with either sulphonlyureas or metformin but not with insulin or 'triple therapy'.

As a precaution it is recommended that liver function tests are performed at baseline and every two months during the first year. Anovulatory women may ovulate if treated with glitazones, so contraceptive advice may therefore be needed.

Repaglinide

Action

Like sulphonlyureas, repaglinide stimulates insulin release. It has a rapid onset of action and a short duration of activity. It is particularly useful in patients who have demonstrated post-prandial peaks (high blood glucose levels $1\frac{1}{2}$–2 hours after food) or in those who have been or who are likely to be hypoglycaemic on sulphonlyureas.

Side-effects

Hypoglycaemia and, more rarely, visual disturbances, abdominal pain, diarrhoea, vomiting, constipation and increase in liver enzymes.

Timing and dose

Repaglinide should be taken before main meals on a 'one meal one dose' basis to accompany between two and four meals a day. Recommended doses are as follows:

If previously on diet alone	0.5 mg per meal
If added to metformin	0.5 mg per meal
If previously treated with sulphonylureas	1 mg per meal

In weeks 2–3 the starting dose may be doubled and it can continue to be doubled every one to two weeks until the blood glucose is controlled or until a maximum dose of 4 mg per meal or 16 mg per day is reached.

Failure of oral agents in the treatment of Type 2 diabetes

It is common to begin tablet treatment with one group of oral agents and gradually to combine these therapies as tolerated. The frequency of secondary tablet failure (failure of tablets after a period of successful control) increases with the duration of the disease. A progressive decline in beta cell function is part of the natural history of Type 2 diabetes; factors such as obesity and insulin resistance may also contribute to the failure of oral agents. It is important that at diagnosis the possibility of insulin injections being needed, either temporarily such as during or post-surgery, or more permanently, is discussed with the patient. Insulin should never be used as a threat and patients need to be reassured that it is the failure of the tablets and not failure on their part that may make insulin necessary.

When to start insulin is often a difficult decision in those with Type 2 diabetes, unless of course they are losing weight dramatically, are severely symptomatic or are planning pregnancy. Twice-daily insulin treatment has been found to result in an average increase of 5 kg in body weight, of which 63 per cent was accounted for by an increase in fat mass (Groop et al., 1989). The dilemma is often, therefore, whether to convert an overweight patient with poor diabetic control with few symptoms on to insulin, thus converting him or her into an even more overweight patient with only a marginal improvement in control of the diabetes.

Box 2.8: Factors to consider when converting to insulin

- What benefits is insulin likely to give to the patient?
- Does the patient have symptoms?
- Has the patient lost weight?
- Does the patient have complications of diabetes?
- Does he or she have recurrent infections or poor healing?
- Is amyotrophy present? (see p. 79)
- Has a proper trial of tablets been given (e.g. taken at correct times and doses)
- How old is the patient?
- How does the patient feel about insulin therapy?

If the patient complains of thirst, polyuria and weight loss, insulin is indicated and is likely to make the patient 'feel better'. Good glycaemic control may delay the progression of complications such as background retinopathy to more serious conditions such as proliferative retinopathy; insulin may therefore be advisable. The presence of renal failure or hepatic insufficiency may make the use of oral agents inadvisable. Amyotrophy may be reversible with insulin and is therefore a clear indication for insulin treatment.

Unfortunately the position is usually less clear cut. The patient has often had poor glycaemic control for a number of years, has tried all available oral agents, is already overweight, is unable to increase exercise and feels only slightly unwell. It is vitally important to involve the patient in the decision and to discuss the likely benefits and disadvantages of insulin. It is important that the patient makes an informed decision. We have found a three-month trial period of insulin useful and this shows patients that we appreciate their opinions and fears (Weedon and Curry, 1992).

Insulin treatment regimes for people with Type 2 diabetes

Groop (1997) cites three options:

- Pre-mixed short- and intermediate-acting insulin, e.g. Mixtard 30 or Humulin M3.
- Multiple injections/basal bolus regime – short-acting insulin before meals and isophane before bed.
- Combination of tablets and insulin, e.g. isophane insulin in the morning or evening with a sulphonylurea or metformin during the day. We have used metformin in addition to twice-daily pre-mixed insulin in patients converted to insulin who are overweight, in an attempt to prevent hyperinsulinaemia.

A once-a-day dose of lente or isophane insulin is rarely sufficient to control blood glucose levels, although it may occasionally be sufficient if symptom control is the only aim of treatment. With the arrival of glargine (see p. 41) a new long-acting analogue once-daily insulin may be possible in those with Type 2. Multiple injections are more likely to encourage weight gain (Yki-Järvinen et al., 1992) and are therefore usually unsuitable for use in those with Type 2 diabetes. A combination of once-daily isophane insulin with daytime sulphonylurea therapy provides comparable short-term blood glucose control to that of twice-daily injections of pre-mixed insulin, but this can rarely be maintained long term (Groop, 1997).

Like Groop (1997), we currently favour twice-daily pre-mixed insulin for those with Type 2 diabetes, via either a syringe or a pen device, or twice-daily isophane such as Humulin I or Human Insulatard, if overweight, transferring to a mixture which incorporates quick-acting insulin if blood glucose levels are unacceptably high before lunch or bed.

Conversion

Conversion to insulin is most successfully undertaken as an outpatient under the supervision of a diabetes specialist nurse (DSN). It is important that the patient has been seen by the dietitian as changes such as snacks may be necessary. Competent home blood glucose monitoring (HBGM) should be ensured. It is vital that the patient has the opportunity to discuss his or her expectations, fears and worries regarding insulin therapy. It is natural for patients to have some concerns and these should be addressed before beginning to teach the mechanics of drawing up insulin. Common fears include needles, hypos, weight gain, eating out and whether they will ever be able to retain the necessary information. The opportunity to talk to others treated with insulin has proved valuable for a number of patients. At Greenwich we have a voluntary patient helper who meets the patient prior to his or her conversion to insulin and is available for 'a chat' on the morning he or she is converted to insulin (Weedon and Curry, 1992; Curry et al., 1993).

Fear of needles is perhaps the quickest worry to allay for the majority of patients. Before the decision to start insulin is made, they should have the opportunity to see the DSN self-inject with an empty insulin syringe and then try it themselves. The majority of injections are painless and patients are normally pleasantly surprised. Hypoglycaemia, its causes and treatment should be discussed prior to conversion and patients reassured that insulin doses will be adjusted slowly according to HBGM readings, taking into account the effects of work and exercise.

The amount of weight which the patient may gain should be discussed with the dietitian and advice given prior to conversion on how to limit this. Weight should be monitored and taken into consideration before insulin doses are increased.

The DVLA issues a three-year licence to car drivers treated with insulin on the condition of a satisfactory medical report. Insulin-treated patients cannot hold heavy goods vehicle (HGV) or public service vehicle (PSV) licences. This may be a problem for those who currently hold these licences. In the past some patients have been able to negotiate with their companies to drive smaller vehicles; for others, insulin treatment has meant loss of job and a career change.

Unfortunately on 1 January 1998 a new Europe-wide directive imposed new driving restrictions on those treated with insulin. Patients treated with insulin will no longer be able to drive vehicles in group C and group D, which were previously covered by a standard UK driving licence. These groups include motor vehicles between 3.5 and 7 tonnes for carrying goods, and passenger vehicles with more than eight seats but fewer than 16. As a result many people with insulin may lose their job when they attempt to renew their driving licence.

It is recommended that patients do not drive for about four weeks after conversion to insulin. Change in blood glucose levels may lead to blurred vision and patients need to know how to prevent, recognize and treat hypoglycaemia.

Reassurance can be given that insulin and food can be safely delayed for a couple of hours if eating out or on holiday. Sport and exercise should be encouraged and the DSN is able to help with adjustments to insulin doses and times.

Only small amounts of information should be given at each visit, which should be revised and built on at subsequent visits. Coles (1991) argues that patients should be helped to relate knowledge to their own situation. Written information should be given reinforcing key points.

A series of appointments as a 'conversion package' are given at Greenwich. Conversions are planned for a Monday morning. The patient arrives at 9 am, having taken no oral hypoglycaemic agents and eaten no breakfast. The patient gives his or her own first insulin injection which the DSN draws up, explaining her actions. The patient then spends the morning in the diabetes centre talking to our patient helper, having breakfast and practising drawing up insulin. Issues such as hypos, storage and timing of insulin and injection sites are discussed and an identification card and dextrose tablets are given for the patient to carry in case of emergency.

The patient is seen the next day at 9 am after having given his or her own evening injection at home. Any problems or difficulties are discussed and the patient has an opportunity to give the morning insulin dose with the support of the nurse. Prevention, recognition and treatment of hypos is revised and reuse of syringes and disposal of sharps discussed. A further appointment is arranged during the first week followed by weekly appointments for the next three weeks. Further appointments are arranged as required. At these visits adjustments to insulin doses are made, how the patient feels and his or her knowledge are evaluated and information such as what to do during intercurrent illness is given. We also offer conversion to insulin in a group setting, again with a series of appointments (see p. 108). The education of patients is covered in detail in Chapter 4.

The following case-studies are intended to help fit the most appropriate treatment to individuals with Type 2 diabetes.

Case-study 2.3

Robin Foster is 40 years old and was diagnosed as having Type 2 diabetes three months ago. He has stopped taking sugar in his tea and coffee and exchanged chocolate bars for fruit. He has also joined the local gym. However, his HBGM results are always above 10 mmol/L even before food, he feels thirsty and needs to get up twice in the night to pass urine. His BMI is 23 and his HbA1$_c$ is 8 per cent (normal range = 3.8–6.2).

What treatment would you advise? What information would you give? I would suggest:

- Start a sulphonylurea. Perhaps gliclazide 80 mg once a day, half an hour before breakfast.
- The dose should be increased according to his HBGM results until blood glucose readings range between 4 and 8 mmol/L most of the time.
- Monitor the effect on weight (BMI should not exceed 25).
- Inform about the risk of hypoglycaemia, and how to prevent, recognize and treat hypos. Discuss the importance of regular meals and the need to decrease the sulphonylurea or increase food prior to exercise in the gym.
- Discuss the effects of alcohol and sulphonylureas.

Case-study 2.4

Margaret Funnell is 58 years old and has had Type 2 diabetes for six years. Her BMI is 40 and her diabetes is poorly controlled. Her blood glucose was 14 mmol/L when checked by the practice nurse. She is treated with glibenclamide 15 mg once a day and has normal renal and hepatic function. Margaret says that she eats very little but that her blood glucose levels and her weight seem to have increased. She 'skips' breakfast in an attempt to reduce calories, has fruit for lunch and a cooked meal in the evening. A 'couple' of times a week Margaret feels faint and dizzy and requires 'a drop' of Lucozade or a bar of chocolate.

What treatment and advice would you give? I would suggest:

- Stop glibenclamide and exchange for metformin 500 mg twice a day.
- Metformin should be taken after food to prevent diarrhoea; it is therefore most important to eat regularly.
- Try to eat three meals a day.
- The faintness and dizziness were likely to be due to hypoglycaemia.
- Hypoglycaemia is not possible with metformin.
- Metformin is likely to encourage weight loss.
- Refer Margaret to a dietitian.

Case-study 2.5

Sidney Pitts is 75 years old and has had Type 2 diabetes for 30 years. He is currently treated with glipizide 10 mg three times a day, metformin 850 mg three times a day and acarbose 100 mg three times a day. Mr Pitts complains of getting up three times in the night to pass urine, lack of energy and an ulcer on his foot which is slow to heal. His BMI is 19 and his $HbA1_c$ is 10.9 per cent. He lives alone, manages his own cooking and shopping but needs a magnifying glass to read.

What treatment does Mr Pitts clearly need? What do you need to assess? I would suggest:

- Mr Pitts needs insulin.

Need to assess:

- His attitude towards insulin. Discuss his anxieties and fears.
- His ability to see the marks on a syringe and ability to draw up insulin. Would he prefer a magnifier or a pen? Is a district nurse required?
- Does Mr Pitts test his own blood glucose? How accurate is his technique? May need to be taught how to perform HBGM or revision of technique. A district nurse may be necessary.
- Does he eat regularly? What and how much?

The Treatment of Type 1 Diabetes

Unlike those with Type 2 diabetes, those with Type 1 diabetes have no available endogenous insulin and without insulin injections they would die. Insulin therapy is therefore necessary in those with Type 1 diabetes. In this section various insulin regimes will be discussed in addition to a brief look at pancreatic and islet cell transplants and the artificial pancreas.

The presentation of Type 1 diabetes and how it can be distinguished from Type 2 diabetes is discussed in Chapter 1 (see p. 9). The management of those with Type 1 diabetes has become a central role of the DSN and providing the patient does not have ketoacidosis, newly diagnosed Type 1 diabetes can be managed on an outpatient basis by the hospital diabetes team. Access to rapid hospital laboratory assistance (blood glucose, electrolytes and bicarbonate estimations) is vital to manage new Type 1 diabetes safely (Grant and Marsden, 1991a). Please see Chapter 4 (p. 109) for a detailed description of the educational management of people with Type 1 diabetes.

The type and dose of insulin used varies according to the needs of the individual and somewhat to the preferences of the health care professionals. Fox and Pickering (1995b) argue that there is no right or wrong way to start insulin. They begin with twice-daily doses of Human Mixtard 30 via a syringe or pen. Other specialists use Humulin I or Human Insulatard or a basal bolus regime. We tend to use three times a day injections of soluble insulin such as Human Actrapid or Humulin S in those with ketones (but not acidosis) for the first day or two and then transfer to whichever regime the patient feels will most suit his or her lifestyle and needs. The benefit of using quick-acting insulin is that the patient feels better and ketones disappear quickly. We feel it is important that the patient begins to feel well before being bombarded with information.

Factors which influence the decision as to which insulin regime to choose include: how the patient feels about injections; shift work; involvement in sport; how regularly the patient eats; how the patient feels about injecting insulin at work; and the preferred method of administration.

Human or animal insulin

Patients are usually commenced on human rather than beef or pork insulin. Patients often need reassurance that this is not derived from 'dead people' and that they cannot contract AIDS from human insulin. Human insulin is genetically engineered from bacteria in a laboratory. The structure of pork insulin differs from human insulin by one amino acid and beef differs from human insulin by three amino acids. In the past beef insulin was reported to cause antibody reactions such as lipoatrophy (a wasting of fat with unsightly hollows at injection sites) and occasionally a local allergy to insulin. These have become extremely rare now human and purified animal insulins are most commonly used. Some patients have recently expressed concern regarding BSE.

Some may have seen television programmes or newspaper articles in the late 1980s and early 1990s about the dangers of human insulin. The Insulin Dependent Diabetes Trust was launched in 1994 as a patient/carer-based organization especially to support those having problems with human insulin. Reported problems which have been attributed by some to human insulin have included hypoglycaemic unawareness, depression, forgetfulness, lack of energy and insomnia. There has been no conclusive proof of the relationship between human insulin and these problems and it remains a controversial issue. Patients' fears and worries should be acknowledged and the facts discussed openly and honestly. If insulin from an animal source is preferred by the patient then it should be used.

Both the Insulin Dependent Diabetes Trust and Diabetes UK have lobbied insulin manufacturers to produce pork and beef insulin cartridges for use in pen injection systems in addition to providing assurance of the continuing production of animal insulins. In 1997 pork and beef insulin cartridges became available and can be used in conjunction with Owen Mumford Autopens.

Types of insulin

The array of different insulin names and different types of pen devices can be confusing and daunting. The types of insulin and regimes most commonly used do, however, fit into clear categories.

(1) Soluble (clear) insulin

This is sometimes known as quick-acting insulin and until recently was the most rapidly acting insulin available. It begins to work after approximately 30 minutes, peaks between two and four hours and lasts for about 6–8 hours.

Table 2.3: Examples and availability of soluble (clear) insulin

Insulin name	Vials	Cartridges	Preloaded pens
Human Actrapid	Yes	Yes (3 ml)	Yes
Humulin S	Yes	Yes (3 ml)	Yes
Pork Actrapid	Yes	No	No
Hypurin Porcine Neutral	Yes	Yes (1.5 ml)	No
Hypurin Bovine Neutral	Yes	Yes (1.5 ml)	No
Insuman Rapid	Yes	Yes (3 ml)	Yes

(2) Quick-acting analogue insulin (clear)

This is a modification of the insulin molecule and is the most rapidly acting insulin currently available. Lispro (Humalog) and insulin aspart (NovoRapid) are the only types of insulin available in this group. The onset of action is approximately 15 minutes and it lasts $3^{1}/_{2}$–4 hours.

(3) Intermediate-acting (cloudy)

(a) Isophane (the most popular type of cloudy insulin). Begins to work after approximately two hours, peaks at 4–12 hours and lasts for about 22–24 hours.

(b) Lente. Starts to work after approximately two hours, peak of action 6–14 hours and lasts for about 22–24 hours.

(4) Long-acting (cloudy)

The peak of action varies from patient to patient and can range from 8–12 hours. Duration can be up to 28 hours.

Table 2.4: Example and availability of analogue insulin

Insulin name	Vials	Cartridges	Preloaded pens
Humalog	Yes	Yes (3 ml)	Yes
NovoRapid	Yes	Yes (3 ml)	Yes

Table 2.5: Examples and availability of isophane insulin

Insulin name	Vials	Cartridges	Preloaded pens
Human Insulatard	Yes	Yes (3 ml)	Yes
Humulin I	Yes	Yes (3 ml)	Yes
Pork Insulatard	Yes	No	No
Hypurin Porcine Isophane	Yes	Yes (1.5 ml and 3 ml)	No
Hypurin Bovine Isophane	Yes	Yes (1.5 ml and 3 ml)	No
Insuman Basal	Yes	Yes (3 ml)	Yes

Table 2.6: Examples and availability of lente insulin

Insulin name	Vials	Cartridges	Preloaded pens
Human Monotard	Yes	No	No
Humulin Lente	Yes	No	No
Hypurin Bovine Lente	Yes	No	No

(5) Long-acting basal (clear)

Insulin Glargine is a new long-lasting insulin analogue which has a prolonged 24-hour absorption profile with no pronounced peaks. It is clear and therefore requires no resuspension, thus eliminating one of the causes of variability in absorption of cloudy medium- and long-acting insulins.

Table 2.7: Examples and availability of glargine (long-acting analogue)

Insulin name	Vials	Cartridges	Preloaded pens
Lantus	Yes	Yes (3ml)	Yes

(6) Pre-mixed (mixtures of soluble, quick-acting analogue and isophane insulin)

The most popular is the 30/70 mixture, 30 per cent soluble and 70 per cent isophane insulin. Humalog Mix 25, Humalog Mix 50 and NovoMix 30 are mixtures of analogue and isophane insulin.

Table 2.8: Examples and availability of long-acting insulin

Insulin name	Vials	Cartridges	Preloaded pens
Human Ultratard	Yes	No	No
Humulin Zn	Yes	No	No
Hypurin Bovine Lente	Yes	No	No
Hypurin Bovine ProtamineZinc	Yes	No	No

Table 2.9: Examples and availability of pre-mixed insulins

Insulin name		Vials	Cartridges	Preloaded pens
Humalog Mix	25	No	Yes (3 ml)	Yes
Humalog Mix	50	No	No	Yes
NovoMix	30	Yes	Yes (3 ml)	Yes
Human Mixtard	30	Yes	Yes (3 ml)	Yes
	10	No	Yes (3 ml)	Yes
	20	No	Yes (3 ml)	Yes
	40	No	Yes (3 ml)	Yes
	50	Yes	Yes (3 ml)	Yes
Humulin	M2	No	Yes (3 ml)	No
	M3	Yes	Yes (3 ml)	Yes
	M5	Yes	No	No
Pork Mixtard	30	Yes	No	No
Hypurin Porcine Biphasic				
Isophane 30/70 Mix		Yes	Yes	No
Insuman Comb	15	Yes	Yes (3 ml)	Yes
Insuman Comb	25	Yes	Yes (3 ml)	Yes
Insuman Comb	50	Yes	Yes (3 ml)	Yes

Cartridges which fit Novopens are called Penfill, e.g. Human Mixtard 20 Penfill; those containing Humulin or Insuman insulin are called Cartridge, e.g. Humulin S Cartridge, Insuman Basal Cartridge, Lentus Cartridge. Preloaded pens are called either Pen, e.g. Human Insulatard Pen; Optiset Pen; Innolet, e.g. Innolet Mixtard 30; Humaject Prefilled Pen, e.g. Humaject M3; or FlexPen, e.g. NovoRapid FlexPen.

Timing of injections

It is recommended that soluble and cloudy insulins are taken 20–30 minutes before a meal. Soluble insulin is most effective in controlling post-prandial hyperglycaemia when taken 30 minutes before food (Gale, 1996). Many patients find this inconvenient, particularly if they are using a basal bolus regime when soluble insulin is required before each meal (three times a day). Many patients therefore ignore this advice and inject immediately before or occasionally after meals. Quick-acting analogue insulin should be taken 5–15 minutes before a meal. In a study, 76 per cent of patients found this more convenient (Gale, 1996).

Insulin regimes

Insulin concentrations in those without diabetes increase sharply in response to meals and return fairly quickly to a lower 'basal' secretion of insulin between meals and during the night. At no point is there no secretion of insulin. Exact insulin requirements are provided which maintain blood glucose levels between narrow limits despite variations in food, exercise and hormone levels. It is difficult to 'mirror' this response. Pancreatic insulin is normally secreted into the portal circulation and only half the amount secreted reaches the systemic circulation.

Those who inject insulin have a low portal level of insulin and a high systemic insulin level, the reverse of 'normal'. Insulin absorption from the tissues is variable and can be influenced by temperature, site of injection, lumps at injection sites and exercise. The amount of insulin is merely a guess at requirements even if diet and exercise remain fairly stable; we have little control over hormone levels, climate and body temperature. The action of manufactured insulin is also imprecise and the duration of action may be different from that required. Snacks between meals are therefore often necessary to prevent hypoglycaemia.

'Insulin is injected in the wrong place, at the wrong time and in the wrong amounts' (Gale, 1996).

Gale (1996) echoes the thoughts of many involved in diabetes care when he claims that it is remarkable that so many people achieve such good control given the crudity of the therapy.

Commonly Used Insulin Regimes

Which insulin regime should be used?

This depends on the needs of the individual and whether tight control (HbA1$_c$ ≤ 7 per cent) is necessary. The risks of hypoglycaemia, which are greater if control is tight (DCCT, 1993), need to be measured against the benefits of tight control and patient preference. It is important to achieve tight control before and during pregnancy (see Chapter 6, p. 167), in those with early complications, and if possible in most young adults. Tight control is unnecessary in those with a limited life expectancy and may be dangerous in those with loss of hypoglycaemic awareness or young children, as hypoglycaemia may impair normal brain development (Gordon and McDowell, 1996).

Once-daily insulin

Once-daily lente or isophane insulin is unlikely to achieve good control and it is obvious from Figure 2.2 (see pp. 46–48) that it does not imitate normal physiology, but it may be useful in the elderly.

However, since the launch of glargine (August 2002) once-daily insulin has become a more effective regime for those with Type 2 diabetes, either used alone or with oral blood glucose-lowering medication. This is because glargine provides a relatively constant basal insulin supply without the peaks of isophane and lente insulins.

Twice-daily regime

This is the most commonly used insulin regime. A mixture of soluble and isophane or lente insulin is injected before breakfast and before the evening meal. The peak of the soluble insulin is unlikely to be sharp enough to prevent hyperglycaemia for the first hour after breakfast and after the evening meal. Soluble insulin lasts too long and its action overlaps with the cloudy insulin; unless snacks are eaten between meals, hypoglycaemia is likely. The peak of the evening cloudy insulin 4–12 hours after it is taken would lead to hypoglycaemia during the night unless a snack is taken before bed.

During pregnancy, when nocturnal hypoglycaemia is common, the evening dose of insulin may be split. The soluble insulin would be given prior to the evening meal and the cloudy insulin before bed; the cloudy insulin therefore peaks before breakfast rather than during the night.

Despite their limitations, twice-daily insulin regimes are favoured by many patients and health care professionals. It is a convenient regime as injections are not required during 'normal' working hours; many people work regular hours and eat regularly. Free mixing rather than a pre-mixed regime is generally recommended for those who have Type 1 diabetes.

Free mixing gives more flexibility for dose adjustment for occasions such as eating out or taking exercise. It is safer for managing intercurrent illness when extra doses of soluble insulin may be needed to prevent or eliminate ketones. The morning and evening doses of cloudy insulin overlap and for this reason it is commonly recommended that they should be injected at regular intervals. As a general rule of thumb patients are advised to inject the morning and evening doses 8–12 hours apart and preferably within about two hours of the 'normal' time. For example, if the evening meal is usually eaten at 7 pm but the patient was eating out at 9 pm the insulin dose could safely be delayed. However, a curry at midnight will require adjustments. For example, the cloudy insulin could be given at the usual time followed by a light snack and the soluble insulin could be given at the restaurant prior to the meal.

Unfortunately, no pen device has been produced which allows clear and cloudy insulins to be free-mixed. Pre-mixed insulins can, however, be used in pens and should be provided for those who prefer them; soluble insulin should also be provided for use in emergencies.

Basal bolus regime (soluble or quick-acting analogue insulin before each meal and intermediate- or long-acting insulin before bed)

A pen device is usually used. The major advantage of this regime is its flexibility. If a meal is delayed the dose of soluble insulin can be delayed and given 20–30 minutes before the meal; quick-acting analogue insulin can be injected immediately before the meal. This regime works well for those who work shifts, eat out regularly and exercise.

A disadvantage of this regime is that patients may be tempted to 'chase their tails'. For example, the before-lunch reading is found to be high, an increased dose of soluble insulin is given to bring it down, and this leads to hypoglycaemia later in the afternoon when the soluble insulin peaks. The evening meal dose of soluble insulin is reduced, causing a rise in blood glucose before bed. The patient is then left with a difficult choice of whether to ignore this or give an extra dose of soluble insulin and continue the process. The correct way to adjust insulin is to wait and look for a pattern. If the blood glucose is regularly high at a certain time of day the insulin dose which peaks at that time of day should be altered. This is the insulin given before and not after the blood glucose reading. For example, a high blood glucose reading before lunch would be affected by the before-breakfast dose of soluble insulin.

Multiple injection regimes have also been associated with high doses of insulin (over-treatment) and weight gain (Jensen et al., 1986, Small et al., 1988). Multiple injection regimes have not been shown to improve diabetic control, although patients often favour them. Hardy et al. (1991) claimed that blood glucose control may deteriorate in young women with diabetes who change to a basal bolus regime using a pen injector.

Pens

There are a large variety of insulin pens available and designs are continuously changing. Any list would therefore soon be outdated. They fall into three main categories:

(1) *Pens which use cartridges.* These are either provided free of charge by the insulin company via diabetes centres, e.g. Humapen Ergo (Eli Lilly), or can be obtained on prescription from the GP, e.g. Novopen 3, BD Pen, Autopen. Novopens use only Novo Nordisk insulins. The pen cartridges and needles

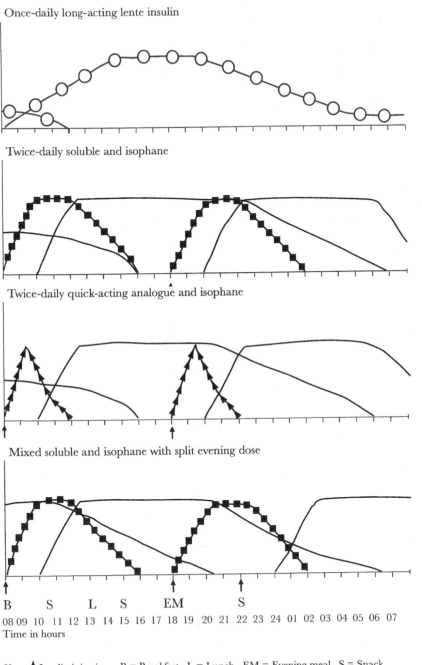

Once-daily long-acting lente insulin

Twice-daily soluble and isophane

Twice-daily quick-acting analogue and isophane

Mixed soluble and isophane with split evening dose

B   S   L   S   EM   S
08 09 10 11 12 13 14 15 16 17 18 19 20 21 22 23 24 01 02 03 04 05 06 07
Time in hours

Key: ↑ Insulin injection   B = Breakfast   L = Lunch   EM = Evening meal   S = Snack

■■ = Soluble insulin   — = Isophane insulin   O-O = Lente insulin   ➤ = Analogue insulin

Figure 2.2: Commonly used insulin regimes

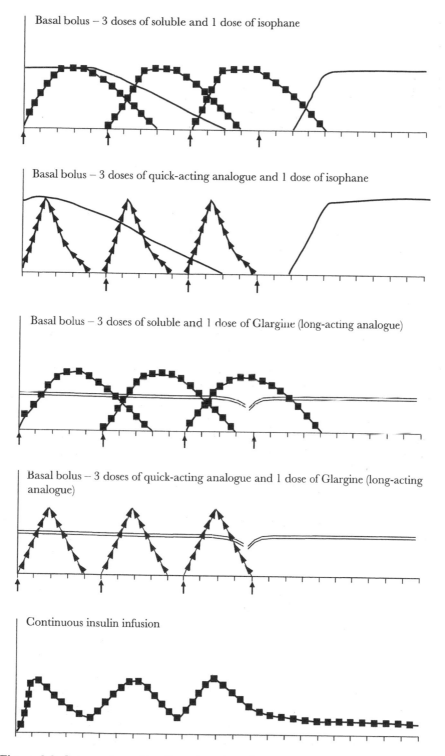

Figure 2.2: Commonly used insulin regimes (contd)

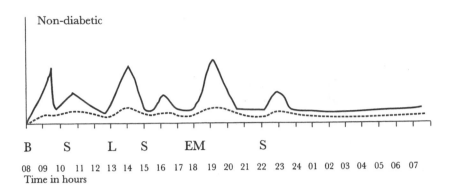

Non-diabetic

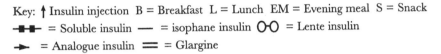

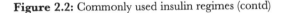

B   S   L   S   EM   S

08 09 10 11 12 13 14 15 16 17 18 19 20 21 22 23 24 01 02 03 04 05 06 07
Time in hours

Key: ↑ Insulin injection B = Breakfast L = Lunch EM = Evening meal S = Snack
━■━ = Soluble insulin ── = isophane insulin O-O = Lente insulin
➤ = Analogue insulin ═ = Glargine

Figure 2.2: Commonly used insulin regimes (contd)

are available on prescription. The pens come in a range of colours and designs and the maximum single dose that can be given varies.

(2) Pre-loaded pens which can be disposed of when empty. These may be easier to use for the elderly or those with poor dexterity who find changing cartridges difficult. Pre-loaded pens are available on prescription. There have recently been two very different disposable pens launched. One is the Innolet (Novo Nordisk). This has a large dial like a kitchen timer, which is easy to turn and depress. The other is the Optiset Pen (Aventis). This allows a carer to set the dose and the patient only has to lift up and press the plunger to deliver repeated set doses until the pen is empty. The original 'Pen' has been updated to a FlexPen, but both remain available at present.

(3) The Innovo insulin doser. This is an insulin adminiatration device (not really a pen at all). Made by Novo Nordisk, it contains an integral battery and has a more stable injection platform than a pen. It has a digital display, which shows the size of the insulin dose, the elapsed time since an injection was last given and a countdown for removal of the needle from the injection site. At present this device is available only through diabetes centres.

Pen needles are available in a range of sizes from 5 mm to 12 mm (see Chapter 4, p. 112 for more information).

Many find pens more discreet, more attractive and therefore more portable, which has helped to remove the embarrassment of injecting insulin in public places. Some types of pen have proved invaluable to patients with poor vision, allowing them to manage their injections independently. Some with poor dexterity may also find pens helpful although they may find the plunger rather stiff to depress, particularly in the case of disposable pens. This can lead to inaccurate dose administration and bruising. Pens are very helpful for many patients but not for all.

Continuous subcutaneous infusion of insulin (CSII)

In theory this regime most closely mimics the normal insulin response to food. A constant infusion of soluble insulin is delivered by a pump attached by fine tubing to a butterfly needle placed under the patient's skin. Extra pulses (amounts) of insulin can be given before each meal. According to Everett and Kerr (2000) only 320 people in the UK compared with 60,000 in the USA and 40,000 in Europe use CSII despite the fact that the Diabetes Control and Complication Trial (1993) found that 42 per cent of the intensified therapy group were using CSII by the end of the study (see p. 60 for more information). Basal bolus regimes have not been found to be universally popular, particularly with teenagers and young adults (Shaw, 1997). Everett and Kerr (2000) claim that pump therapy reduces hypoglycaemia, aids the return of warning signs of hypos, and allows hourly insulin adjustment, flexible eating patterns and injections only every 2–3 days.

On the negative side, they are expensive. Pumps cost around £2000 and infusion sets, cartridges and batteries cost around £15 per week. The external pump is a visible reminder of diabetes 23 hours a day, carbohydrate intake needs to be closely monitored and blood glucose measurements need to be performed frequently. Also, insulin syringes or pens must always be carried to prevent ketoacidosis due to pump failure.

Adjustment of insulin doses

As a DSN I am keen to teach patients how to adjust their own doses of insulin and thus encourage independence. However, some patients continue to see insulin adjustment as the job of health care professionals and are therefore reluctant to self-adjust insulin. Gill and Redmond (1991) found that, even amongst interested and motivated patients, knowledge of how to adjust insulin doses safely is poor. Interestingly it was the basal bolus system which seemed to cause the most confusion. Gill and Redmond (1991) argue that self-adjustment skills need to be specifically taught to selected patients and their response evaluated. They argue that for most patients it may be 'prudent to opt for a passive clinic based dose adjustment policy'.

I feel that all patients should be given an opportunity to learn insulin adjustment and therefore to take control of their diabetes. If patients prefer not to, or are unable to take responsibility for dose adjustment, they should be reassured that the DSN/doctor is happy to change insulin doses and will not put them under pressure to self-adjust.

For some patients only small or infrequent adjustments are necessary, for example during hot weather, gardening or illness. For others, shift work or regular travel that crosses time zones may make it vital that patients are able to self-adjust insulin doses. In order to change doses safely, accurate blood glucose measurements are needed at varied times of the day. It is most helpful if these are written in a diary.

Colours or shapes drawn in the blood testing diary can be used to help patients understand the effects of each dose of insulin at particular times of the day. Other patients prefer diagrams or lists. It is important to ask patients what they prefer.

Except in the case of illness (see p. 134) patients should be advised to wait for a pattern to emerge before changing insulin doses. They should also be taught to look at diet and injection sites (lumpy sites may affect control) before assuming that the insulin dose is at fault. Cloudy insulin should not be changed more frequently than every 2–3 days. Cloudy insulins taken twice daily overlap in effect and more frequent adjustments may lead to hyper- or hypoglycaemia. Patients should be taught to work backwards from the high or low blood glucose and therefore treat the cause rather than the symptom of the problem. As discussed on p. 45, there is a temptation to give more or less insulin at the time of one high or low blood glucose level and 'chase the tail'.

It is important that insulin injections should *never* be withheld even if the blood glucose level is too low. The 'hypo' should be treated and then the insulin given as usual. It is not the insulin that is about to be given that caused the hypo but the dose which has already been given. It is therefore the previous insulin dose or dietary behaviour which requires adjustment.

Patients can be set small tasks for which insulin doses require adjustment, based on activities in which the patient would like to participate – for example, a late night meal, swimming, etc. Results can be discussed and feedback given by the DSN. It is an excellent way to apply theory to practice and make advice relevant to individuals.

Pancreatic and Islet Cell Transplants

Patients often ask about transplants. Pancreas transplants are performed in Britain in specialist centres. The main problem is that immunosuppression is required which carries numerous risks including infection, malignancy and diabetes itself. At the present time pancreas transplants are usually restricted to people who require renal transplants and would therefore require immunosuppression anyway. The outcome of pancreas transplants is disappointing: approximately 30–35 per cent fail in the first year and 50 per cent by five years (Abecassis and Corry, 1993; Sutherland, 1992).

It is suggested that in the future immunosuppression may not be necessary for islet cell transplants. There may be potential to coat the cells with a neutral substance, or to make cells neutral by using multiple cell culture to breed out their genetic expression (Burden, 1991). It is unlikely that enough human islet cells would be available so the use of pig cells has been suggested. London et al. (1991) feel that if advances in technology continue, islet cell transplantation as treatment for Type 1 diabetes is achievable. It is, however, likely to take some time.

In May 2000 *The Guardian*, *The Times*, *The Telegraph* and the *Daily Mail* carried the story of the work of James Shapiro, a surgeon who has successfully transplanted islet cells into eight people with previously poorly controlled diabetes. At one year post surgery 100 per cent of the transplants were successful. Diabetes UK (2000) acknowledged this as 'a real breakthrough' but are cautious and have highlighted a number of issues which require consideration before the treatment becomes widely available.

(1) Risk of transplant procedure. It is currently only offered to people with tremendous difficulty controlling diabetes conventionally and who are therefore at huge risk of ketoacidosis, complications and poor quality of life.
(2) Long-term anti-rejection therapy drugs are necessary. One of them, sirolimus (Rapamune) is not yet licensed in the UK and only licensed in the USA and Canada for renal transplants. The long-term effects are unknown.
(3) Problem of supply and demand. Each patient received 12,000 islet cells per kilogram of their body weight. For each transplant the islet cells of two donor pancreases were needed. There is already a severe shortage of donor organs for established transplant procedures.

Inhaled Insulin

Inhaled insulin is currently undergoing phase III trials and may be available in the UK in a few years. The devices are similar to inhalers used for treating asthma and use compressed air to deliver tiny particules of insulin into the lungs, from where the insulin enters the bloodstream.

The Mechanical Pancreas

A mechanical implantable pancreas requires miniaturization and coordination of an insulin pump, a glucose sensor and a control system (e.g. alarms for hypo/hyperglycaemia). Thompson et al. (1998) have described the successful use of such devices in the management of Type 2 diabetes.

National Service Framework

The NSF standards relevant to this chapter are shown in Box 2.9.

Questions (one for each learning outcome)

(1) You have been asked to write some simple dietary advice for a patient with newly diagnosed diabetes, who will not see the dietitian until next week. He is anxious and unable to take in too much information. What advice would you include?
(2) You have been asked to discuss briefly the benefits and disadvantages of various therapies used to treat Type 2 diabetes. What would you include?
(3) Sam is 23 years old and he was diagnosed with Type 2 diabetes two days ago. He is currently taking Actrapid 6 units three times a day and he would like information on which insulin regime to use on a more long-term basis. He eats regularly, works on a building site and plays football on a Sunday morning. What would you advise?

Suggested answers are found on pages 249–51.

Box 2.9: NSF standards

Standard 3: Empowering people with diabetes
(3) All children, young people and adults with diabetes will receive a service which encourages partnership in decision-making, supports them in managing their diabetes and helps them to adopt and maintain a healthy lifestyle. This will be reflected in an agreed and shared care plan in an appropriate format and language. Where appropriate, parents and carers should be fully engaged in this process.

Standard 4: Clinical care of adults with diabetes
(4) All adults with diabetes will receive high-quality care throughout their lifetime, including support to optimize the control of their blood glucose, blood pressure and other risk factors for developing the complications of diabetes.

Standards 5 and 6: Clinical care of children and young people with diabetes
(5) All children and young people with diabetes will receive consistently high-quality care and they, with their families and others involved in their day-to-day care, will be supported to optimize the control of their blood glucose and their physical, psychological, intellectual, educational and social development.

(6) All young people with diabetes will experience a smooth transition of care from paediatric diabetes services to adult diabetes services, whether hospital or community based, either directly or via a young people's clinic. The transition will be organized in partnership with each individual and at an age appropriate to and agreed with them.

References

Abecassis M, Corry RJ (1993) An update on pancreas transplantation. Advances in Surgery 26: 163–88.

British Diabetic Association (1996–7a) Balance for Beginners – Starting Out with Non Insulin Dependent Diabetes. London: BDA, pp 44–6.

British Diabetic Association (1996–7b) Sick Days Balance For Beginners – Starting out with Insulin Dependent Diabetes. London: BDA, pp 88–9.

Burden AC (1991) Human islet transplantation – the way ahead. Practical Diabetes 8(3): 81.

Chan AW, MacFarlane IA (1988) The pharmacology of oral agents used to treat diabetes mellitus. Practical Diabetes 5(2): 59–64.

Clarke BF, Campbell IW (1977) Comparison of metformin and chlorpropamide in non-obese maturity onset diabetes uncontrolled by diet. British Medical Journal 275: 1576–8.

Coles C (1991) Diabetes education; theories of practice. Practical Diabetes 6(5): 199–202.

Curry M, Weedon L, Marsden P (1993) Patient helpers – the forgotten resource. Practical Diabetes 10(3).

Department of Health (1991) National Framework for Diabetes Standards. London: HMSO.

Department of Health (1994) Committee on Medical Aspects of Food Policy. National Aspects of Cardiovascular Disease. London: HMSO.

Diabetes Control and Complication Trial Research Group (1993) The effect of intensive treatment of diabetes on the development and progression of long-term complications in insulin-dependent diabetes mellitus. New England Journal of Medicine 329: 977–86.

Diabetes UK (2000) Behind the headlines. Balance. September–October 2000. London: Diabetes UK, pp. 20–22.

Everett J, Kerr D (2000) Insulin pump therapy: a fresh start for the UK. Journal of Diabetes Nursing 4(2): 44–7.

Fox C, Pickering A (1995a) Diabetes in the Real World. London: Class Publishing, pp 61–78.

Fox C, Pickering A (1995b) Treatment of insulin dependent diabetes mellitus. In Diabetes in the Real World. London: Class, pp 45–59.

Frost G, Wilding J,Beecham J (1994) Dietary advice based on the glycaemic index improves dietary profile and metabolic control in Type 2 diabetic patients. Diabetic Medicine 11: 397–401.

Fuessl HS, Williams G, Adrian TE, Bloom SR (1987) Guar sprinkled on food: effect on glycaemic control, plasma lipids and gut hormones in non-insulin-dependent patients. Diabetic Medicine 4: 463–8.

Gale EAM (1996) Insulin lispro: the first insulin analogue to reach the market. Practical Diabetes International 13(4): 122–4.

Garrow JS, Owens AM (1990) Dietary fibre, food intake and obesity. In Bloom SR (Ed) Fibre – Is It Good For You? Southampton: Duphar Medical Relations, pp 37–48.

Gill GV, Redmond S (1991) Self-adjustment of insulin: an educational failure? Practical Diabetes 8(4): 142–3.

Gordon J (1996) Dietary advice. In McDowell JRS, Gordon D (Eds) Diabetes – Caring for Patients in the Community. Edinburgh: Churchill Livingstone, pp 109–31.

Gordon D, McDowell J (1996) The patient with insulin dependent diabetes mellitus. In McDowell JRS, Gordon D (Eds) Diabetes: Caring for Patients in the Community. Edinburgh: Churchill Livingstone, pp 81–107.

Grant J, Marsden P (1991a) Module 5 Initiating Insulin therapy. In Diabetes Care in General Practice. Basingstoke: Eli Lilly, p 13.

Grant J, Marsden P (1991b) Module 3 Oral hypoglycaemic therapy. In Diabetes Care in General Practice. Basingstoke: Eli Lilly, pp 3–17.

Groop LC (1997) Drug treatment of non-insulin-dependent diabetes mellitus. In Pickup J, Williams G (Eds) Textbook of Diabetes. 2nd edn. Oxford: Blackwell Science, pp 38.1–38.18.

Groop LC, Widen E, Franssila-Kallunki A, Eastrand A, Salorant C, Senalin C, Eriksson J (1989) Different effects of insulin and oral anti diabetic agents on glucose and energy metabolism in type 2 (non-insulin dependent) diabetes mellitus. Diabetologia 32: 599–605.

Ha T, Lean MEJ (1997) Diet and lifestyle modification in the management of non-insulin dependent diabetes mellitus. In Pickup J, Williams G (Eds) Textbook of Diabetes. 2nd edn. Oxford: Blackwell Science, pp 37.1–37.18.

Hardy KJ, Jones KE, Gill GV (1991) Deterioration in blood glucose control in females with diabetes changed to a basal-bolus regime using a pen injector. Diabetic Medicine 8: 69–71.

Health Education Authority (1996) Think About Drink (Education leaflet). London: HEA.

Hoechst (2001) Summary of Product Characteristics – Amaryl. Uxbridge: Hoechst Marion Roussel Ltd, p. 7.

Jenkins DJA, Wolever TMS, Vuksen et al. (1989) Nibbling versus gorging: metabolic advantages of increased meal frequency. New England Journal of Medicine 321: 929–34.

Jensen T, Moller L, Andersen O (1986) Metabolic control and patient acceptability of multiple insulin injections using Novopen cartridge packed insulin. Practical Diabetes 3: 302–6.

Lean MEJ, Brenchley S, Connor H, Elkeles RS, Govindji A, Martland BV, Lord K,

Southgate DAT, Thomas BJ (The Nutrition Subcommittee of the British Diabetic Association's Professional Advisory Committee) (1992) Dietary recommendations for people with diabetes: an update for the 1990s. Diabetic Medicine 9: 189–202.

London NJM, James RFL, Bell PRF (1991) Advances in human islet cell transplantation. Practical Diabetes 8(3): 96–8.

Melander A, Bitze'n PO, Faber O, Groop L (1989) Sulphonlyurea antidiabetic drugs: an update of their clinical pharmacology and rational therapeutic use. Drugs 37: 58–72.

National Institute for Clinical Excellence (2000) Guidance on Rosiglitazone for Type 2 Diabetes Mellitus. Technology Appraisal Guidance No 9. August 2000. London: NICE.

National Institute for Clinical Excellence (2001) Guidance on Pioglitazone for Type 2 Diabetes Mellitus. Technology Appraisal Guidance No 21. March 2001. London: NICE.

Nutrition Study Group of the European Association for the Study of Diabetes (1988) Nutritional recommendations for individuals with diabetes mellitus. Diabetes Nutrition and Metabolism 1: 145–9.

Shaw KM (1997) Insulin lispro: insulin with a rapid onset of action. The Prescriber 19 February.

Small M, MacRury S, Boal A, Paterson KR, MacCuish AC (1988) Comparison of conventional twice daily subcutaneous insulin administration and multiple injection regimen (using the novopen) in insulin-dependent diabetes mellitus. Diabetes Research 8: 85–9.

Stumvoll M, Nurjhan N, Perriello G, Dailey G, Gerian JE (1995) Metabolic effects of metformin in non insulin dependent diabetes mellitus. New England Journal of Medicine 333: 550–4.

Sutherland DER (1992) Pancreatic transplantation: state of the art. Transplantation Proceedings 24: 762–6.

Swedish Diabetic Association (1987) Kost and Diabetes. Stockholm: Svenska Diabetes Forbundet.

Thomas BJ and The Nutrition Subcommittee of the Professional Advisory Committee of the British Diabetic Association (1992) Discussion paper on the role of diabetic foods. Diabetic Medicine 9: 300–6.

Thompson JS, Duckworth WC, Saudek CD, Giobbie-Hurder A (1998) Surgical experience with implantable insulin pumps. Department of Veterans Affairs Implantable Insulin Pump Study Group. American Journal of Surgery 176: 622–6.

United Kingdom Prospective Diabetes Study Group (UKPDS) 13 (1995) Relative efficacy of randomly allocated diet sulphonylureas insulin or metformin in patients with newly diagnosed non-insulin dependent diabetes followed for 3 years. British Medical Journal 310: 83–8.

Weedon L, Curry M (1992) Switching to insulin. Nursing Times 88(49): 34–6.

Wolever TMS (1997) The glycaemic index: flogging a dead horse? Diabetes Care 20: 452–6.

Wu M-S, Johnston P, Shen WH-H, Hollenbeck LB, Jeng LY, Goldfine ID, Chew YD, Reavon GM (1990) Effect of metformin on carbohydrate and lipoprotein metabolism in NIDD patients. Diabetes Care 13: 1–8.

Yki-Järvinen H, Kauppila M, Kaujansuu E, Lanti J, Tapawi M, Niskanen L, Rajala S, Ryysy L, Salo S, Seppala P, Tvlokas T, Karjaiaven J, Taskinen MB (1992) Comparison of insulin regimes in patients with non-insulin-dependent diabetes mellitus. New England Journal of Medicine 327: 1426–33.

Zeller K, Whittaker E, Sullivan L, Raskin P, Jacobsen HR (1991) Effect of restricting dietary protein on the progression of renal failure in patients with insulin-dependent diabetes mellitus. New England Journal of Medicine 324: 78–84.

Chapter 3
The complications of diabetes

This chapter addresses both the acute complications and the long-term complications of diabetes. The acute complications discussed are diabetic ketoacidosis and hyper-osmolar non-ketotic syndrome. The long-term complications are divided into microvascular and macrovascular complications. The causes, diagnosis and management of complications are examined.

Learning Outcomes

By the end of this chapter you should be able to:

(1) Safely recognize and manage diabetic ketoacidosis and hyper-osmolar non-ketotic coma.
(2) Suggest to patients with both Type 1 diabetes and Type 2 diabetes ways to reduce the risk of long-term complications of diabetes.
(3) Provide likely reasons for erectile dysfunction in men with diabetes. Discuss investigations that will be necessary and the treatment options available.

Acute Complications of Diabetes

Diabetic ketoacidosis (DKA)

Alberti (1974) defines DKA as 'severe uncontrolled diabetes requiring emergency treatment with insulin and emergency fluids with a blood ketone body concentration of greater than 5 mmol/L' (p. 68). As most hospitals do not have access to blood ketone measurements, urinary ketones are usually measured using dipsticks such as Ketostix. Medisense now produce an optium sensor for patient use which allows blood ketone testing in addition to blood glucose testing. The company recommend patients to contact a health professional if the β-ketone test result is greater than 1.5 mmol/L (mid-range). It is hoped that the optium will soon be available for hospital ward/department use. Krentz and Nattress (1997) define the diagnostic criteria as a capillary or arterial plasma bicarbonate of 15 mmol/L or less, with urine Ketostix of ++ or more.

Hurel et al. (1997) claim that DKA is the largest single cause of death in patients with diabetes under the age of 40 years. They estimate mortality rates to range between 2 per cent and 22 per cent. Rates are particularly high in the elderly and in those with other medical illnesses. Gale et al. (1981) claim that rates are also higher in less specialized centres.

Causes of ketoacidosis

Box 3.1: Precipitating factors in DKA

(1) Infection – found to be the commonest identifiable cause by Krentz and Nattress (1997) and Hurel et al. (1997)
(2) New presentation of Type 1 diabetes
(3) Mismanagement of diabetes by either patient or health professional. Hurel et al. (1997) found that of 23 patients in whom infection precipitated DKA, 10 had omitted their insulin
(4) No obvious cause

The mismanagement of diabetes may be an educational problem (see Chapter 5 for management of intercurrent illness) or due to psychosocial or psychiatric problems. Hurel et al. (1997) claim that at least one-third of patients with DKA have problems with personality or compliance and social, domestic or psychiatric problems.

Box 3.2: Clinical features of DKA

Thirst, polyuria, nocturia, blurred vision, leg cramps, weight loss, generalized weakness, facial flushing, deep rapid breathing (Kussmaul respiration), nausea, vomiting, abdominal pain, drowsiness and, if untreated, coma

---

The symptoms of DKA usually develop quickly over a period of days rather than weeks. It is often vomiting which leads to hospital admission. Patients with severe DKA have signs of dehydration, hypotension and tachycardia.

Diagnosis

A finger-prick blood glucose measurement and urine dipstick capillary blood test for ketones should be performed immediately in the accident and emergency department and treatment should be initiated on the basis of these. Venous blood should then be taken for urgent laboratory measurement of glucose, urea, electrolytes, bicarbonate and full blood count. Arterial pH and bicarbonate should also be measured to confirm the diagnosis. Urine, blood and sputum should also be sent for culture if infection is suspected. A chest X-ray and ECG, cardiac enzymes and amylase should be performed as clinically indicated. A history should be taken to try to ascertain the cause.

Box 3.3: Aims of treatment

(1) To rehydrate the patient and correct the deficit of sodium and potassium and the acidosis
(2) To decrease blood glucose levels to 10 mmol/L or less within 24 hours
(3) To correct hypotension

Cautions

Abdominal pain may be misdiagnosed. Plasma amylase levels can often be raised in ketoacidosis (Warshaw et al., 1977). Many people are unable to smell ketones, therefore absence of ketones on the breath cannot be relied upon. Peripheral vasodilatation may lead to hypothermia, thus preventing a rise in body temperature to indicate underlying infection. Conversely, a rise in neutrophil count may occur in DKA without infection. Plasma potassium concentration may be temporarily raised despite severe intracellular depletion.

The precise management of DKA will depend on the protocol of the hospital in which you work, and the age of the patient. The following guidelines are broadly followed in most units.

Fluid and electrolytes

- Intravenous 0.9 per cent normal saline 1000–1500 ml in 1 hour and 500–1000 ml in each of the next four hours. The rate of administration and the total quantity of fluid are dependent on the severity of dehydration and the age of the patient. Caution is needed in the elderly and in those with heart failure.
- No potassium is added to the first 500–1000 ml of saline but 20–40 mmol of KCl may be added to the next litre bag, dependent on plasma potassium levels.
- When blood glucose is reduced to 10–15 mmol/L, 5 per cent dextrose should be used rather than saline.

Insulin

- Insulin is usually given intravenously by continuous insulin syringe pump, 1 unit/per ml. Soluble insulin such as Actrapid, Velosulin or Humulin S is used. A rate of 6 units per hour is given initially and increased or decreased according to blood glucose levels. The insulin pump should not be turned off until subcutaneous insulin has been given. The patient with DKA has insulin-dependent diabetes and therefore requires exogenous insulin. If blood glucose levels are less than 4 mmol/L the rate or concentration of the glucose infusion or the rate of the insulin pump requires review by the medical team.
- Once blood glucose has been reduced to 10–15 mmol/L, 5 per cent dextrose should be given at about 150 ml per hour until the patient is able to eat normally.

- When the patient is able to eat, electrolytes are normal and blood glucose levels are less than 15 mmol/L, subcutaneous insulin should be given. This should be given 1 hour before the intravenous insulin is stopped to allow absorption from the subcutaneous fat, and 30 minutes before a meal.
- Frequent estimations of electrolytes are necessary. Potassium levels should be checked two-hourly (Krentz and Nattress, 1997).
- Urine output should be measured and accurate fluid balance charts kept.
- Hourly estimations of blood glucose using a blood glucose meter are necessary while intravenous insulin and glucose are administered. Insulin doses should be adjusted according to the results. It is important that the blood glucose monitoring is performed accurately. The finger used must be washed with soap and water (a flannel can be used for this purpose). If the finger has glucose or fruit juice on it the measurement obtained will reflect the amount of sugar on the finger rather than in the patient's bloodstream.
- The insulin infusion rate and the blood glucose level should be recorded on the same chart. Insulin and glucose delivery lines should be checked for blockages and the working of the pump checked if blood glucose levels are not falling.
- A nasogastric tube should be inserted if the patient is unconscious, because of the risk of aspiration of stomach contents.
- A urinary catheter should be passed if the patient is unconscious or has not passed urine within four hours of admission (Krentz and Nattress, 1997). A urinary catheter increases the risk of infection and is unpleasant for the patient.
- The monitoring of central venous pressure may be necessary for those who are elderly or in heart failure.

The use of bicarbonate to treat DKA is controversial. Hypokalaemia, impaired myocardial contractability and overshoot alkalosis are all potentially dangerous effects of bicarbonate administration. Thrombosis of the vein into which bicarbonate is given may occur and extensive local necrosis may be caused by extravasation. Bicarbonate is therefore usually given only if the patient is severely acidotic or if cardiorespiratory collapse is imminent (Krentz and Nattress, 1997).

Complications of DKA

These include: (1) cerebral oedema, which is rare in adults and is poorly understood; (2) adult respiratory distress syndrome, which may require intermittent positive pressure ventilation; and (3) thromboembolic complications such as venous thrombosis, stroke and, rarely, disseminated intravascular coagulation.

Hyper-osmolar non-ketotic syndrome (HONK)

HONK is characterized by marked hyperglycaemia which may exceed 60 mmol/L without significant ketonuria and acidosis. Patients are often severely dehydrated and uraemic and are often drowsy. The onset of hyperglycaemia develops over weeks rather than hours or days in the case of DKA.

HONK usually affects middle-aged or elderly patients. Up to 60 per cent of those affected have previously undiagnosed diabetes (Lewis et al., 1996). Mortality is high at over 30 per cent (Krentz and Nattress, 1997) and thromboembolic complications are common.

Causes

HONK may be precipitated by infection, treatment with antihypertensive agents such as thiazide diuretics and a large intake of glucose drinks.

Diagnosis

This is confirmed by marked hyperglycaemia and increased plasma osmolarity in the absence of ketosis and acidosis.

Box 3.4: The differential diagnosis of DKA and HONK

HONK	DKA
Often found to have a high plasma sodium concentration	Plasma sodium concentration usually normal or low
Blood glucose > 50 mmol/L	Blood glucose may be only slightly elevated and usually less than 40 mmol/L
Negative or small quantities of ketones in the urine/blood	Moderate or large ketones in urine/blood
Plasma bicarbonate usually 18 mmol/L or above	Low plasma bicarbonate usually less than 15 mmol/L
Slow onset of hyperglycaemic symptoms (weeks)	Quick onset of diabetic symptoms (days)
Symptoms rarely include vomiting. No Kussmaul respirations	Symptoms may include vomiting and Kussmaul respirations
If previously undiagnosed with diabetes the patient is likely to be middle aged or elderly	If previously undiagnosed with diabetes the patient is most likely to be (but not exclusively) under 30 years old

---

Management of HONK

Emergency. The initial management is the same as for DKA. Intravenous insulin is used. Hypotonic (0.45 per cent) saline rather than isotonic (0.9 per cent) saline is used if plasma sodium is elevated. Heparin 24,000 units IV should be given in 24 hours due to the high risk of thromboembolic complications.

Longer term. As in the case of DKA, subcutaneous insulin should be given when the patient is able to eat normally. Subcutaneous insulin is usually continued for about three months. After this it is usually possible for patients to be controlled on a diet or oral hypoglycaemic agents.

Chronic Complications of Diabetes

Both Type 2 diabetes and Type 1 diabetes can result in macrovascular and microvascular complications. Microvascular (small blood vessel) complications affect the eyes (retinopathy), the kidneys (nephropathy) and the nerves (neuropathy). Macrovascular (large blood vessel) complications are caused by reduced blood flow to the tissues because of atherosclerosis. These complications include angina, myocardial infarction, cerebrovascular accidents and amputations.

The incidence and progression of complications vary in Type 2 and Type 1 diabetes. The diagnosis of Type 2 diabetes may be delayed owing to the absence of symptoms. According to Marks (1996) the United Kingdom Prospective Diabetes Study (UKPDS) found that half of those newly diagnosed with Type 2 diabetes had one or more microvascular or macrovascular complications. If hypertension and impotence are included as complications then 65–75 per cent had complications at diagnosis.

The length of time that a person has diabetes and the level of glycaemic control during this period have been associated with the severity of microvascular complications (Pirart, 1978). The longer the person has diabetes and the poorer the level of glycaemic control the greater the risk of the development and progression of retinopathy, neuropathy and nephropathy. It is, however, important to note that not all people with poor glycaemic control who have had diabetes for a long time develop complications. Factors such as age, sex, race, ethnicity, socioeconomic status, hypertension, hyperlipidaemia and smoking have been implicated (Herman and Crofford, 1997). I shall now discuss the evidence that supports the relationship between glycaemic control and diabetic complications and the implications of these findings.

Hyperglycaemia: its Relationship to Diabetic Complications

The Diabetes Control and Complications Trial (DCCT)

The American Diabetes Association (ADA, 1993) described the DCCT as a 'landmark multi-center trial' which has both statistical and clinical significance. It found that lowering blood glucose concentration slows or prevents the development of diabetic complications.

The DCCT asked two related questions:

(1) Could intensive therapy and 'tight' control prevent the development of diabetic retinopathy in patients with no retinopathy? (primary prevention).
(2) Could intensive therapy and 'tight' control slow the progression of early retinopathy? (secondary intervention).

Description of the study

Subjects who participated in the DCCT had Type 1 diabetes. A total of 1441 patients between the ages of 13 and 39 years were recruited between 1983 and 1989. The study ended in 1993 after an average follow up of 6.5 years (range 3–9 years).

A total of 726 patients were in the primary prevention group and 715 patients were in the secondary intervention group. Patients in each group were randomly allocated to either intensive (tight) or standard (conventional) treatment. Intensive therapy involved insulin injections three or more times a day or continuous subcutaneous insulin infusion (CSII), intensive education about diet and insulin adjustment, self-monitoring of blood four or more times a day, weekly telephone calls and monthly clinic visits. Conventional treatment involved one or two insulin injections a day, clinic visits every three months and an education programme. This type of management did not include or encourage adjustments to the insulin dose in response to self-monitoring data (Herman and Crofford, 1997).

Level of glycaemic control achieved

At the beginning of the study the mean $HbA1_c$ (glycated haemoglobin) was approximately 8.9 per cent. At about six months the $HbA1_c$ of those receiving intensive therapy improved and a significant difference in mean $HbA1_c$ between intensively and conventionally treated groups was maintained. Those assigned to the conventional treatment group maintained $HbA1_c$ values of about 9 per cent. Those in the intensive treatment group maintained $HbA1_c$ values of about 7 per cent.

Results

Box 3.5: Reduction of complications in the intensively controlled primary prevention group	
Complication	Reduction when compared with conventionally treated group (%)
Retinopathy (from 5 years onwards)	76
Neuropathy (from 5 years)	69
Nephropathy (measured by microalbuminuria)	34

Box 3.6: Reduction in complications in the intensively controlled secondary intervention group

Complications	Reduction when compared with the conventionally treated group (%)
*Retinopathy (after 3 years)	54
Neuropathy (after 5 years)	57
Nephropathy (as measured by microalbuminuria)	43

---

*Note: During the first year those receiving intensive therapy had a higher incidence of retinopathy than those in the conventionally treated group. However, after this a progressive benefit was found in the intensively treated group.

Intensive therapy (tight control) was found to be effective in both delaying the onset and slowing the progression of early retinopathy, neuropathy and nephropathy.

Side-effects of intensive treatment/tight control

Despite the advantages of intense treatment with regard to long-term complications, there are important disadvantages to tight control. In the intensively treated group there were 62 severe hypoglycaemic episodes per 100 patient years which required help from others, compared with 19 in the conventional therapy group. There were 16 episodes per 100 patient years in the intensively treated group compared with five who were given conventional treatment. Hospitalization rates for hypos were 54 and 36 in the intensively treated and conventionally treated groups respectively. There were 12.7 cases of obesity reported in the intensive treatment group and 9.3 cases in the conventional therapy group. The ADA (1993) acknowledges this weight gain as significant and accepts the adverse medical and emotional problems that it may cause.

Limitations of the DCCT

The patients selected for the study were not representative of the general population with Type 1 diabetes. Fox and Pickering (1995) describe how participants were carefully selected using stringent practical and psychological tests. Patients were highly motivated, young and generally healthy. The professional personnel carrying out the study were trained endocrinologists and diabetes educators working in centres of excellence. Fox and Pickering (1995) claim that the extra resources required (such as the time of health professionals) to support intensively treating patients to this level in the UK would total an extra £720 per patient per year.

Intensified treatment makes more demands on the patient, his or her family and health care professionals. British Diabetic Association (1993) recommend that the DCCT should not be used as a stick with which to bully and frighten people. The conclusions of the DCCT study group suggest that intensified insulin regimes are necessary. Many patients are not keen on the idea of three or four injections a day, preferring two.

Perhaps further research is needed to answer the following questions: Can tight glycaemic control be achieved using two insulin injections a day? Was it the number of insulin injections or the level of professional support and education which improved glycaemic control, or a combination of factors?

The DCCT was designed to determine the effects of tight control on microvascular rather than macrovascular disease. The young age of the participants meant that large vessel disease was too rare to detect significant differences in outcome between the two treatment groups.

The United Kingdom Prospective Diabetes Study (UKPDS)

The UKPDS was designed to find out whether improved glycaemic control helps to prevent complications in patients with newly diagnosed Type 2 diabetes. It also examined the effects of different treatment regimes. The trial began in 1977 and by March 1991 it included 5100 patients in 23 centres in England, Scotland and Northern Ireland. Unlike the DCCT, the UKPDS recruited a representative sample of people with Type 2 diabetes.

All patients were treated with diet for four months. Those with a fasting blood glucose greater than 6 mmol/l after this period were randomized to either diet treatment alone, treatment with sulphonylureas or insulin. Patients who were overweight were randomized to metformin treatment. Patients in whom treatment with sulphonylureas or metformin alone failed were further randomized to combination therapy (treatment with both metformin and sulphonylureas). Those who developed symptoms of hyperglycaemia or a high fasting blood glucose on maximal oral therapy were transferred to insulin.

Importantly, 39 per cent of patients entering the study were found to be hypertensive (BP > 160/90 mmHg or > 150/85 on anti-hypertensive therapy), a hypertensive arm was therefore added (UKPDS, 1998b), to examine whether tighter blood pressure control would reduce the risk of microvascular and macrovascular complications. This study examined whether treatment with beta-blockers or angiotensin-converting enzyme (ACE) inhibitors had specific advantages or disadvantages.

The UKPDS found that intensive blood glucose control substantially reduced the risk of some microvascular but not macrovascular disease. Although the $HbA1_c$ in the more intensively treated group was only 1 per cent lower over 10 years than in the group treated conventionally, this improvement was associated with a 25 per cent reduction in the risk of microvascular complications and a 12 per cent reduction in the risk of any diabetes-related endpoint. Sulphonylureas and insulin were equally effective in reducing $HbA1_c$.

The only therapy shown to reduce macrovascular complications was metformin in overweight patients, with a significant reduction in diabetes-related deaths, all-cause mortality and myocardial infarction (UKPDS, 1998c). The addition of metformin to sulphonylurea therapy showed a significant increase in diabetes-related deaths. The study investigators acknowledge that this requires further study but attribute it to fewer than expected deaths in the sulphonylurea-alone group and the short follow-up period. There is felt to be no indication to stop combined metformin-sulphonylurea therapy (Campbell, 1999).

Tight control of blood pressure (144/82 mmHg) gave significant benefit with regard to micro- and macrovascular complications. This included reduction in progression of retinopathy (34 per cent), a 37 per cent reduction of microvascular endpoints, a 44 per cent reduction in the risk of strokes and a 56 per cent reduction in heart failure. Tight BP control in hypertensive patients reduced the risk of any microvascular or macrovascular diabetes–related endpoint by 24 per cent compared with the 12 per cent reduction obtained by improved glycaemic control. Of particular significance was that tight blood pressure control slows the development of maculopathy where glucose control does not. The ACE inhibitor captopril and the beta blocker atenolol were found to be equally effective. After six years 28 per cent of subjects required three or more drugs to achieve tight blood pressure control.

Perhaps the most striking findings of the UKPDS are the relentless progressive nature of Type 2 diabetes (the median $HbA1_c$ of 7 per cent in the early years rose to 8.2 per cent at 10 years despite intensive efforts to normalize blood glucose) and that up to 50 per cent of patients with newly diagnosed diabetes showed signs of diabetic complications. The UKPDS demonstrated that blood glucose control will not significantly alter macrovascular complications. Correction of other factors – obesity, hypertension, dislipidaemia and smoking – is necessary in the management of Type 2 diabetes.

A questionnaire survey with the UKPDS found that intensive management of glycaemia and hypertension did not affect the overall quality of life (except for those with frequent hypoglycaemia). Patients who required laser treatment for retinopathy had an increased incidence of mood disturbance and tension, and those who suffered myocardial infarction or stroke reported significant reduction in mobility and vigour. The message appeared clear – complications reduce the quality of life; therapy to prevent complications does not.

Based on the UKPDS findings, approximately 600,000 patients in the UK are in need of additional oral medication and/or insulin treatment, as well as closer follow-up and more frequent review (Gallichan, 1999).

The UKPDS demonstrated that the costs of additional medication for improving blood glucose control were offset by lower costs for hospital admissions. Intensive control increased treatment costs by an average of £695 per patient, but reduced the cost of complications by £957 (UKPDS, 1998d). Achieving good control also requires more visits to health care providers and thus additional staff costs. Despite this, the overall cost effectiveness compares favourably with other accepted uses of health care resources.

Limitations of the UKPDS

Despite the peak incidence of Type 2 diabetes occurring between 65 and 69 years in men and 70 and 74 years in women (Stout, 1991) the patients recruited to the UKPDS were aged between 25 and 65 years with a mean age of 53 years. There is therefore no concrete evidence that the benefits of improved BP and blood glucose control seen in the younger minority of patients will apply to the older majority of patients with Type 2 diabetes. Since the UKPDS study began, newer, shorter acting sulphonylureas such as gliclazide have largely superseded glibenclamide and chlorpropamide. We do not know whether these drugs have the same effects.

As in the DCCT, patients in the intensively treated group of the UKPDS reported more hypoglycaemic episodes and weight gain was significantly higher. Those assigned to insulin had the greatest weight gain. This highlights again the cost of tight control to patients and the importance of patient involvement in treatment decisions.

The importance of post-prandial glycaemia

It is now clear that fasting glucose concentrations alone do not identify individuals at increased risk of death associated with hyperglycaemia.

A number of studies have identified a strong correlation between post-prandial hyperglycaemia and cardiovascular death. These studies include the Hoorn Study (De Vegt et al., 1999), the Honolulu Heart Study (Donahue et al., 1987), the Chicago Heart Study (Lowe et al., 1997) and the DECODE Study (1999). The DECODE study, which involved over 25,000 with a mean follow up of 7.3 years, indicated that an increased mortality risk was associated with two-hour postload plasma glucose levels to a much greater extent than fasting plasma glucose.

The St Vincent Declaration

The World Health Organisation, the International Diabetes Federation, patient organizations (including the BDA) and government health representatives from all European countries signed the St Vincent Declaration in 1989.

General goals and five-year targets were set in an effort to reduce the morbidity and mortality associated with diabetes. Issues such as education of patients, their friends and work associates in addition to professional education are addressed. Independence, equity and self-sufficiency for all people with diabetes are promoted together with the removal of hindrances which exist preventing the full integration of the person with diabetes into society. Some may therefore question the appropriateness of driving legislation (1998) (see p. 116). The setting up of quality assurance schemes and European and international collaboration are recommended.

The section most relevant to this chapter is that which aims to implement effective measures for the prevention of serious and costly complications:

- reduce cases of new blindness by one-third or more
- reduce numbers of people entering end-stage renal failure by at least one-third
- reduce by one-half the rate of limb amputations for diabetic gangrene
- cut morbidity and mortality from coronary heart disease in the diabetic by vigorous programmes of risk factor reduction
- achieve pregnancy outcome in the diabetic woman that approaches that of non-diabetic women.

In the next section I shall examine microvascular and macrovascular complications of diabetes. Complications will be defined, risk factors identified, and prevention, screening procedures and treatment will be discussed.

Microvascular Disease

Retinopathy

Diabetic retinopathy is a disease of the small blood vessels in the retina. In those with Type 1 diabetes and Type 2 diabetes retinopathy progresses in slightly different ways. This will be discussed later. Diabetic retinopathy is the most common cause of visual loss in the working population (Grey et al., 1989), accounting for 20 per cent of registrations for blindness in the 16–65 year age-group. Approximately 2 per cent of the diabetic population become blind and this figure is expected to fall as a result of screening and laser treatment (Fox and Pickering, 1995). The actual prevalence and incidence of blindness in the UK are not known. Bruce et al. (1991) argue that only approximately one-third of eligible patients are registered as blind. It will therefore be difficult to determine whether the targets of St Vincent are met.

Retinopathy rarely occurs until diabetes has been present for more than five years, but will be evident in almost all people who have had diabetes for over 20 years. It is important to mention again that there may be a delay in the diagnosis of Type 2 diabetes and that retinopathy may therefore be present at diagnosis.

Cataract is approximately five times more common in people with diabetes than in the general population and tends to occur at an earlier age in those with diabetes. Glaucoma is also more common in those with diabetes.

Risk factors and prevention

The prevalence and severity of retinopathy are dependent on the length of time that the patient has had the disease (Klein et al., 1984a). In the Wisconsin Studies Klein et al. (1984b) found in those diagnosed at less than 30 years old that higher age at diagnosis, poor glycaemic control, higher diastolic blood pressure and proteinuria were all high risk factors. For the older group, poor glycaemic control, high systolic blood pressure, proteinuria and the requirement for insulin were risk factors.

The DCCT showed the effect of improved glycaemic control in reducing the incidence and progression of retinopathy in those with Type 1 diabetes (see p. 60). However, the Steno Study Group (1982) claim that the achievement of 'tight control' after a period of poor control in the presence of retinopathy may lead to a deterioration of retinopathy. After two years, vision was found to be similar whether control was tightened or not. The DCCT also demonstrated an improvement in retinopathy after an initial period of deterioration in the intensively treated group. The UKPDS has also indicated that strict blood glucose control reduces the risk of retinopathy and its progression. Reducing blood pressure in hypertensive Type 2 patients has also been shown to reduce the incidence and progression of retinopathy.

Background or non-proliferative retinopathy

In background retinopathy the small blood vessels of the retina become blocked and other vessels dilate in order to compensate.

Background retinopathy in itself is not a threat to vision and does not require laser treatment. Symptoms are not apparent to the patient. Signs in the eye include scattered capillary microaneurysms, followed by small 'dot and blot' haemorrhages and the occasional hard exudate. The retinal vessels become abnormally permeable and leak serous fluid, which leads to the formation of hard exudates. Pre-proliferative changes are recognized by the appearance of cotton wool spots and IRMA (intra-retinal microvascular anomalies).

Proliferative retinopathy

This is sight threatening. Proliferative disease is characterized by the development of new blood vessels in response to ischaemia. New vessels bleed easily, which may lead to a haemorrhage into the vitreous body (jelly of the eye). New vessels can also result in scar tissue which can lead to detachment of the retina. Proliferative retinopathy can lead to sudden and painless loss of vision. If untreated by laser, 60 per cent of eyes will become blind within 5 years (Marks, 1996).

Maculopathy

This is the other sight-threatening form of diabetic retinopathy and it endangers central vision. Maculopathy is preceded by the appearance of hard exudate in patches or rings, forming between the temporal vessels and approaching the fovea. These rings have oedema at their centre (Kohner et al., 1996).

Maculopathy is less common in people with Type 1 diabetes than in those with Type 2 diabetes. When it does occur in Type 1 diabetes it is more likely to be associated with proliferative retinopathy (Herman et al., 1983).

Retinal disease in those with Type 2 diabetes usually starts with hard exudates and microaneurysms which may intensify around the macula, causing a progressive reduction in visual acuity. Early referral is indicated while vision is retained.

Advanced or end-stage disease

Traction on new vessels caused by contraction of fibrous bands may cause shearing leading to haemorrhage into the vitreous body or between the vitreous body and the retina. The patient may notice 'floaters' (black specks travelling across the eye) or major loss of vision. Opaque fibrous tissue also increases traction on the retina, which may detach. If the fovea is involved vision is lost. Vision may have been totally normal prior to this event. Ocular ischaemia is associated with the development of new vessels on the iris. These may obstruct drainage and cause painful thrombotic glaucoma. Advanced retinopathy is sometimes treatable with vitrectomy.

The management of diabetic retinopathy is based on screening and early treatment by laser. These will now be discussed.

Screening

Rohan et al. (1989) claim that a systematic screening programme would prevent about 260 cases of blindness per year in England and Wales. Kohner et al. (1996) challenge this figure, claiming that it assumes 100 per cent patient compliance and an unrealistic involvement of optometrists (87 per cent). Despite these reservations they acknowledge that studies in the USA and the UK indicate that screening for diabetic retinopathy achieves worthwhile health gains.

What Diabetes Care to Expect is a leaflet produced by Diabetes UK for patients and is free of charge. This 'patient's charter' recommends that everyone with diabetes should have their eyes 'checked' every year. According to Kohner et al. (1996) there is no hard evidence to support the optimum time for screening, although yearly is felt to be easiest to administer. For some patients, such as those with Type 1 diabetes who have been diagnosed for less than 5 years, the interval could be longer; in others it should be shorter. All patients should have their eyes examined at diagnosis; this is particularly important in those with Type 2 diabetes who may have significant retinopathy at diagnosis.

Methods of screening

Visual acuity. To test visual acuity a well-lit Snellen chart and a 6-metre distance for the patient to stand at are required. It is possible to use a half-size chart where a distance of 3 metres is required. Fox and Pickering (1995) argue that this is difficult to organize. Kohner et al. (1996) go further, suggesting that in most cases GP practice premises are inadequate for screening for retinopathy either by visual acuity testing or fundoscopy.

If visual acuity is to be checked, patients need to bring their glasses if they are worn for distance reading. If these are forgotten a pinhole should be used to correct the refractive error. The right eye should be checked first, with the left covered with a card. The lowest line read is recorded, for example 6/9. If the line is not complete the letters missed can be recorded, for example 6/9 −3 if three letters were missed. The reading 6/9 means that the patient sees at 6 metres what someone with normal vision would see at 9 metres.

Non-mydriatic camera. This may be situated at a hospital or the camera taken round the community in a mobile clinic. There are concerns about its sensitivity if used alone and the use of mydriatic drops to dilate the eye has been suggested. A benefit of this system is that it provides a permanent record.

Ophthalmoscopy/fundoscopy. This is examination of the eye using an ophthalmoscope. Mydriatic eye drops such as tropicamide 1 per cent should be used. Patients should be advised that these drops may sting and vision may be blurred for 2–3 hours, making driving unsafe.

Ophthalmoscopy may be undertaken by doctors in the hospital clinic, GPs, optometrists and more rarely nurse practitioners or diabetes specialist nurses (DSNs). Fox (Fox and Pickering, 1995) suggests that nurses may become good at ophthalmoscopy, overcoming the problems of GPs who are not keen to examine the fundus! Whether busy practice nurses or DSNs would consider this to be an appropriate use of their time and educational and psychosocial skills is debatable. Retinal photography has been shown to be more effective than conventional ophthalmoscopy. Failure to diagnose proliferative diabetic retinopathy by ophthalmoscopy in the hospital diabetic clinic ranges from 30 to 50 per cent. Retinal photography using Polaroid prints or colour transparancies has been shown to be accurate and sensitive in 96.5 per cent of cases (Nathan et al., 1991; Valez et al., 1987).

The UK National Screening Committee (2000) recommend digital photography as the best retinopathy screening tool. This is because photographs of the retina can be stored on CD-ROM for audit and training purposes. The National Service Framework Delivery Strategy (DoH, 2003) promises capital funds to support the purchase of digital cameras and has identified a UK National Screening Committee to set quality standards, monitory criteria and specifications for information and professional development resources.

Kohner et al. (1996) highlight the lack of training in ophthalmology in most medical schools. They argue that new graduates and GPs with no special training cannot be expected to be competent ophthalmoscopists. More training is therefore necessary. Kohner et al. (1996) argue that if districts believe that the best strategy is for GPs or optometrists to undertake screening, then it is the responsibility of the local ophthalmic consultants to organize training.

The success of any screening programme depends on a good recall system and on the accessibility of the system to the patients. There are a number of patients unable to get to the hospital or optician, such as the housebound. Those who work may find an out-of-hours service more accessible.

Nurses need to be fully aware of the screening system in their district in order to ensure that patients are accessing appropriate care. Patients require education about the importance of screening (see p. 130). O'Hare et al. (1996) emphasize the advantages of using both ophthalmoscopy and retinal photography in the same patients and the use of an ophthalmologist to read the pictures to improve sensitivity. Dilating the pupils using mydriatic fundus photography has also been shown to improve sensitivity (Jones et al., 1988). Patients found to have retinopathy on screening should be referred to an ophthalmologist.

Fox and Pickering (1995) claim that there are three reasons why screening may fail to detect diabetic retinopathy:

(1) Failure of the observer or the camera to identify the problem. This may be due to failure to dilate the eyes fully, or obscured view due to cataract. Rarely there may be disease on the periphery of the retina which is outside the view of the camera.
(2) Rapid deterioration before the time of the next planned screening. Those with active retinopathy should be screened six-monthly. Both pregnancy and a sudden dramatic improvement in diabetic control can lead to deterioration of retinopathy. Fox and Pickering (1995) argue that in these circumstances eyes should be examined every two months.
(3) Failure of patients to attend screening. Patients need to be reminded to attend and to be educated about the importance of attending. A well-organized communication system between primary and secondary care could highlight those who fail to attend and ensure that they are followed up.

Treatment

Laser treatment is an effective treatment for diabetic retinopathy. Kohner et al. (1996) claim that early treatment with laser photocoagulation can prevent blindness in 90 per cent of patients with proliferative retinopathy if applied adequately. Photocoagulation has also been shown to be effective in preventing visual loss due to maculopathy, although treatment is most effective before visual symptoms occur (MacCuish, 1992). This again highlights the importance of an organized retinal screening programme.

What happens during laser treatment should be carefully explained to the patient. Mydriatic drops (to dilate pupils) and anaesthetic drops (so that the contact lens used to focus the laser beam can be tolerated) are required. A bright flash will occur which may be painful to some patients, particularly if a number of sessions have been necessary.

Vitreous surgery may be needed for end-stage disease. Removal of the vitreous body may be effective in improving vision in those with vitreous haemorrhage.

Low-vision clinics should be available to all visually handicapped people, although access to these takes too long and follow-up is not always provided (Kohner et al., 1996). Aids and education can be given to help patients to live as independently as possible.

Nephropathy

Nathan (1993) claims that nephropathy is the diabetes-specific complication associated with the greatest mortality. Mortality is largely associated with uraemia and associated cardiovascular disease. Nephropathy is closely linked to retinopathy. Two-thirds of those with proliferative retinopathy will also have nephropathy (Marks, 1996). In diabetic nephropathy the small vessels in the kidneys become abnormal and protein leaks into the urine. Initially the protein loss is below the level which is detectable by routine 'dipstick' testing for albumin. This stage is called microalbuminuria. Later the protein loss gets bigger and is detectable by Albustix. This stage is called proteinuria. Persistent proteinuria indicates overt nephropathy.

Diabetic nephropathy develops in about 30–35 per cent of those with Type 1 diabetes (Viberti et al., 1996; Trevison et al., 1997). The risk of nephropathy in those with Type 2 diabetes varies according to ethnic origin: 25 per cent of those of European origin compared with around 50 per cent in those of Afro-Caribbean, Asian, Indian and Japanese origin with Type 2 diabetes develop nephropathy (Viberti et al., 1996).

Both those with Type 1 diabetes and those with Type 2 diabetes are at risk of diabetic nephropathy. The disease has a number of stages: microalbuminuria, proteinuria, uraemia and end-stage renal failure. At an early stage (microalbuminuria) most renal changes can be reversed (Viberti et al., 1996).

Screening for diabetic nephropathy

Diabetes UK's 'patient's charter' *What Diabetes Care to Expect* advises patients that they should have their urine tested yearly for protein. No mention is made of testing for microalbuminuria. The presence of microalbuminuria in both Type 1 diabetes and Type 2 diabetes is predictive of persistent proteinuria and early death from cardiovascular disease. Microalbuminuria is also associated with a higher prevalence of retinopathy (particularly in Type 1 diabetes), peripheral vascular disease and neuropathy (Viberti et al., 1996).

Microalbuminuria indicates renal damage at a reversible stage but the evidence for this reversibility is stronger in Type 1 diabetes than in Type 2 diabetes. Patients with Type 1 diabetes and microalbuminuria carry a twentyfold greater risk of developing renal failure than those with Type 1 diabetes without microalbuminuria (Fox and Pickering, 1995).

Viberti et al. (1996) define microalbuminuria as a persistent increase (two out of three consecutive sterile timed urine specimens) in the albumin secretion rate: 20–200 μg per minute or 30–300 mg/day. A timed urine collection either overnight or for 24 hours is often impractical. Viberti et al. (1996) claim that a reliable screening method is to measure albumin concentration or albumin/creatinine ratio in the first morning sample. Dipsticks such as Micral (BM) and Microbumintest (Bayer) have been developed to test albumin concentration in the microalbuminuria range. Viberti et al. (1996) claim that results should be confirmed by quantitative assays.

Fox and Pickering (1995) argue that because of the implications of a positive test (increased risk of renal failure and cardiovascular disease) patients should be given information and emotional support, allowing them to decide whether or not they wish to be tested. A positive result will put them under pressure to take an angiotensin-converting enzyme (ACE) inhibitor (irrespective of blood pressure levels) and to improve diabetic control. However, as these interventions may prevent renal failure most seem keen to be screened.

Patients who develop persistent proteinuria, defined by Viberti et al. (1996) as an albumin excretion rate > 200 μg per minute (300 mg per day), should be monitored three times a year (Viberti et al., 1996). Progression of proteinuria should be checked using either timed urine collections or by early morning albumin/creatinine ratios. Arterial hypertension may occur and excessive protein loss can lead to nephrotic syndrome. Lipid disturbances, atherosclerotic complications and retinopathy are common. Medical assessment for retinopathy, neuropathy and cardiovascular disease is necessary.

Treatment/prevention

Microalbuminuria stage

Blood glucose control should be improved, although uncertainty exists as to whether improved glycaemic control delays progression to proteinuria (Microalbuminuria Collaborative Study Group, 1995).

Blood pressure. Hypertension should be treated. Treatment with ACE inhibitors has been found to delay progression to nephropathy in normotensive people with diabetes (Viberti et al., 1994).

Smoking. Smoking is associated with the development of microalbuminuria. Patients need to be educated about the effects of smoking and given encouragement and support to stop.

Protein restriction. Diets rich in animal protein have been implicated in the development of microalbuminuria in Type 1 diabetes. Although this is not yet proved, Viberti et al. (1996) support a replacement of some animal protein with vegetable protein and a restriction of protein to approximately 0.8–1 g per kg body weight per day.

Lipids. Attempts should be made to lower cholesterol and triglycerides with diet, weight decrease, improved glycaemic control and lipid-lowering agents as necessary. Both micro- and macroalbuminuria increase cholesterol levels, which may explain the high rate of cardiovascular disease.

Proteinuria stage

Blood pressure. Once proteinuria has appeared, renal disease is established and there is a steady progression to end-stage renal failure (ESRF) (Fox and Pickering, 1995). The rate of decline varies and this can be slowed with effective control of blood pressure. Pharmacological intervention is usually necessary. Drugs, including beta-blockers, diuretics, hydralazine and ACE inhibitors, have all been shown to slow the rate of decline in renal function (Viberti et al., 1996). Adding ACE inhibitors to treatment appears to be particularly beneficial in those with Type 1 diabetes (Lewis et al., 1993).

Blood glucose control. There is no evidence that 'tight' control slows the progression of established renal disease. In those with Type 2 diabetes with impaired renal function, metformin, chlorpropamide and glibenclamide should be avoided. Insulin should be used as necessary in those with Type 2 diabetes.

Protein restriction. Protein restriction has been shown to be beneficial in those with Type 1 diabetes with nephropathy (Walker et al., 1989). Protein restriction and the replacement of animal with vegetable protein should be undertaken under the supervision and with the support of a state-registered dietitian.

Serum lipids. Management should be the same as for microalbuminuria.

Serum calcium. This should be checked in patients with proteinuria and raised creatinine. If calcium levels fall, vitamin D treatment for renal bone disease should be considered.

Referral to nephrologists. Viberti et al. (1996) suggest that when serum creatinine levels reach 200 μmol/L referral to renal specialists should be considered.

Patients with renal failure approach the prospect of ESRF and renal replacement therapy or transplant. Psychological support and education will be required. Ideally a joint diabetes/renal clinic should be attended, although these are rare except in specialist centres. Stable glucose control may be more difficult to achieve in insulin-treated patients with renal failure. Insulin is partly metabolized by the kidneys and therefore duration of action may be more variable. Patients in renal failure may require a reduction in insulin dose of up to 50 per cent.

End-stage renal failure (ESRF)

Diabetes no longer excludes patients from renal replacement therapy.

Haemodialysis. Haemodialysis remains the most common form of treatment for people with diabetes with ESRF (Grenfell, 1997). Unfortunately, those with ESRF due to diabetes usually have other problems such as heart disease and severe retinopathy. The formation of fistulas and shunts may be made more difficult by atheromatous peripheral vessels and dialysis may be complicated by postural hypotension and fluid retention.

Continuous ambulatory peritoneal dialysis (CAPD). CAPD avoids rapid volume fluctuations and the need for vascular access and is therefore suitable for the elderly and those with ischaemic heart disease.

Transplants. Grenfell (1997) cites renal transplantation from a live related donor as the treatment of choice in patients under the age of 60. Survival at five years is cited as 80 per cent for live related grafts and 65 per cent in cadavers. In some cases combined kidney and pancreas transplantation (from cadavers) may be considered to maintain normoglycaemia and prevent nephropathy in the transplanted kidney.

Neuropathy

Neuropathy refers to nerve damage; it is a common complication of diabetes and has a vast number of clinical presentations (Clarke and Lee, 1995). Diabetic neuropathy may be associated with autonomic dysfunction, may affect single nerves such as the third cranial nerve or the femoral nerve (amyotrophy) and can increase risk of pressure palsies, for example of the median nerve (carpal tunnel syndrome). Diabetic neuropathy constitutes a diverse group of clinical disorders in which severity ranges from minimal symptoms to devastating and debilitating pain and loss of function.

The prevalence and severity of neuropathy increase with the degree and duration of hyperglycaemia. Neuropathy has been traditionally classed as a microvascular disease (as in this chapter) although evidence from the UKPDS suggests that both microvascular and macrovascular disease contribute.

The mechanisms causing nerve damage are not clearly understood. Metabolic and vascular factors may contribute. Hyperglycaemia is known to be important; both the DCCT and UKPDS demonstrated that tight control decreased the occurrence of clinical neuropathy. Sorbitol and fructose are derived from excess serum glucose, accumulate within the nerve and are associated with increased polyol pathway activity. This may deplete glutathione levels, which are important in protecting the nerve against the effects of free radicals. Nitric oxide production is reduced; this can impair nerve blood flow and lead to enhanced glycation and damage to neural proteins. Aldose reductase inhibitors block polyol pathways and have been shown to improve peripheral nerve function in animals. Benefits to humans have been disappointing (Ward and Tesfaye, 1997).

Impaired blood supply to the nerves may also contribute to peripheral neuropathy.

Watkins and Edmonds (1997) classify neuropathies into three main groups:

(1) Those which progress steadily with increasing duration of diabetes and are associated with other complications of diabetes. Examples include distal symmetrical neuropathy, small-fibre neuropathies such as Charcot joint, autonomic neuropathy.
(2) Abrupt in onset, often occurring at diagnosis of diabetes unrelated to disease duration or other complications of diabetes. Expected to resolve completely. Examples include acute diffuse painful neuropathy and mononeuropathies such as amyotrophy.
(3) Pressure palsies – not specific to diabetes but more common in diabetes, for example carpal tunnel syndrome.

Distal symmetrical neuropathy

This is the most common form of diabetic neuropathy. Nerve loss is not uniform; both myelinated and unmyelinated fibres are damaged, which causes a reduction in the perception of pain and temperature followed by a decline in autonomic nerve function (Guy et al.,1985). Symptomatic autonomic neuropathy is rare. Muscle wasting and weakness due to motor damage are also rare, although asymptomatic motor nerve abnormalities are commonly present. The term 'sensorimotor' is therefore often used.

Distal symmetrical neuropathy usually affects the feet in a stocking distribution. It is often symptomless, causing reduced pain sensation and putting the feet at risk of injury and tissue damage. Some patients may complain of numbness, coldness or 'pins and needles' in their feet. Patients may also complain of contact sensitivity (allodynia), particularly at night with bed covers.

Pain can be severe and may persist for years, although the most severe usually recover within 12 to 18 months. Young (1997) claims that the mechanisms involved in neuropathic pain are controversial. Distal symmetrical neuropathy has a gradual onset and worsens with increased duration of diabetes. The small-fibre neuropathy present progresses to cause symptomatic autonomic neuropathy.

Screening and diagnosis

- *Patient history.* A history of numbness, 'pins and needles' pain or allodynia in a symmetrical stocking distribution may be present, although many patients are asymptomatic.
- *Physical examination.* Examination of sensation and other aspects of neural function.
   (1) Loss of pinprick, light touch, temperature and vibration sensation may be present.
   (2) The reflexes may be absent.
   (3) There may be a loss of sweating in the feet.
   (4) There may be postural hypotension or impotence, indicating autonomic damage.
  (5) Fundi, blood pressure and urinary albumin excretion should be examined to identify other complications which could influence the treatment of neuropathy.

Management

```
Box 3.7: The management of diabetic neuropathy

(1)  Primary preventive measures which slow degeneration of nerve function
(2)  Treatment for specific problems of neuropathy, e.g. pain, oedema
(3)  Secondary prevention of foot ulcers, e.g. patient education, suitable shoes.
     (see p. 128).
```

(1) Primary prevention

Glycaemic control should be tight (see DCCT and UKPDS results). The use of aldose reductase inhibitors and evening primrose oil is under investigation. Vasodilator drugs have been shown to improve nerve function in animals and some are promising in clinical trials (Young, 1997).

(2) Treatment for specific problems of neuropathy

Each patient needs to be listened to and the cause of pain investigated, and other causes of pain such as lumbar disc prolapse excluded. Neuropathic pain is often worse at night. Patient fears and beliefs about their pain require exploration. Guilt regarding poor glycaemic control, anger or fear of amputation will all require sensitive counselling (see Chapter 7).

Patients should be reassured that acute presentations of pain associated with poor glycaemic control and weight loss, or which have occurred after a sudden improvement in diabetic control, will spontaneously abate (Young et al., 1988). Improvement in glycaemic control is considered good practice although there is no evidence to support the idea that improving control improves pain.

Allodynia may accompany burning pain. Treatment usually involves careful choice of clothing next to the skin, a bed cradle, or Opsite applied to the skin. Opsite film applied to the skin has been shown by Foster et al. (1994) to relieve pain associated with diabetic neuropathy. The most likely explanation for its effectiveness is that it may act as a protective barrier to painful stimuli. It may also act in a similar way to transcutaneous nerve stimulation or have a placebo effect. It is not effective in all patients but Foster et al. (1994) recommend that it should be tried before pharmacological treatments with their associated side-effects are used.

The type of drugs used to treat painful neuropathy will depend on the type of pain experienced. Burning pain is most effectively controlled by the use of tricyclic antidepressants. These are thought to relieve pain by blocking nor-adrenaline re-uptake rather than by altering the patient's mood. Amitriptyline is an example of this type of drug. They are usually used at night when neuropathic pain is typically worse, and they can provide sedation. Gabapentin may be used as an alternative to tricyclic anti-depressants. Topical capsaicin, the active ingredient in hot peppers, has also been used (Clarke and Lee, 1995).

Electric-shock-type pains may respond best to anticonvulsant drugs such as carbamazepine. Restless legs may benefit from low-dose clonazepam treatment. Cramp can be effectively treated by quinine sulphate.

(3) The secondary prevention of foot ulcers

Please see pp. 88–93 for a full discussion.

Diffuse small-fibre neuropathy

This is a distinct syndrome in which selective damage is caused to small nerve fibres, leading to severe sensory and autonomic loss. It is most common in young women with Type 1 diabetes. Patients develop severe symptomatic autonomic neuropathy. Unlike other forms of diabetic neuropathy, it is thought to have an autoimmune cause.

Diagnosis

There is loss of thermal sensation and pain. Patients do not, however, experience numbness in the feet, and normal light touch and virtually normal vibration perception is retained.

Treatment/management

The symptoms are treated in a similar way to autonomic neuropathy. The management of Charcot joint is discussed on p. 93.

Autonomic neuropathy

Marks (1996) claims that the figures indicating the prevalence of autonomic neuropathy are vague. Ewing and Clarke (1986) estimate that between 17 per cent and 40 per cent of people with diabetes have autonomic neuropathy. It may affect numerous organs in patients with long-standing diabetes and may often occur at a sub-clinical level (Fox and Pickering, 1995).

Symptoms/diagnosis

(1) *Gustatory sweating.* This is the most common symptom. Sweating begins soon after chewing tasty food, in particular cheese. It starts on the forehead and spreads to the face, neck, scalp and sometimes the chest.
(2) *Postural hypotension.* Symptoms range from mild dizziness on standing to loss of consciousness. Symptoms are usually worse at night. Diagnosis is made by measuring the blood pressure lying and then after standing for two minutes (Watkins and Edmonds, 1997).
(3) *Diarrhoea.* This is relatively uncommon. Causes have been attributed to abnormalities of gut motility, bacterial overgrowth and bile salt malabsorption. Faecal incontinence may be due to the dysfunction of the internal and external sphincters. Abdominal pain and wind may be followed by watery diarrhoea. This commonly occurs at night with faecal incontinence. Episodes are intermittent, with normal bowel habits or constipation between attacks.
(4) *Impotence.* This is relatively common and is discussed on pp. 79–83.
(5) *Cardiovascular changes.* These rarely cause symptoms and include changes in heart rate responses to manoeuvres such as standing, deep breathing and sustained hand grip.
(6) *Diabetic gastroparesis.* This can cause vomiting and regurgitation of food. The diagnosis may be difficult and may require endoscopy, demonstrating a large food residue in the stomach, absent peristalsis and an open pylorus.
(7) *Neuropathic bladder.* The sacral nerves are affected leading to bladder dysfunction. Symptoms are rare but patients may notice a poor stream of urine and overflow incontinence. Bladder emptying may feel inadequate to

the patient. Men with neuropathic bladder function are also impotent. Disorders of the prostate and other causes of obstruction should be excluded and the presence of other features of autonomic neuropathy should be present before a diagnosis of neurogenic bladder is made.

(8) *Respiratory arrests.* Arrests usually follow general anaesthetics or powerful analgesics. There have, however, been reports of patients dying at night with no convincing explanation (Ewing et al., 1980).

(9) *Sub-clinical abnormalities.* These include abnormal pupillary reflexes, oesophageal dysfunction, blunted counter-regulatory responses to hypoglycaemia and increased peripheral blood flow to the feet.

Treatment/management

(1) *Gustatory sweating.* Unfortunately no effective treatments have been found in which benefits outweigh side-effects. The anticholingeric drug poldine has been used but is rarely tolerated because of its tendency to cause urinary retention, tachycardia and dryness of the mouth (Young, 1997).

(2) *Postural hypotension.* Patients should be advised to get out of bed slowly and to exercise leg muscles before standing. Elevation of the head of the bed whilst sleeping and the wearing of elastic tights is also reported to be helpful (Clarke and Lee, 1995). Anti-hypertensive drugs should be avoided and diabetes control improved to avoid dehydration (Watkins and Edmonds, 1997). The use of fludrocortisone is recommended (Fox and Pickering, 1995). Doses of up to 100 μg/day may be necessary (Young, 1997).

(3) *Diarrhoea.* Diarrhoea can often be managed with codeine phosphate or loperamide. Diarrhoea due to bacterial overgrowth can be improved using 3–5 day courses of a broad-spectrum antibiotic.

(4) *Impotence* (see p. 79).

(5) *Cardiovascular changes.* These are sub-clinical and are therefore not treated.

(6) *Gastroparesis.* Poor glycaemic control has been shown to delay gastric emptying (Fraser et al., 1990). Metoclopramide, domperidone and cisapride are all useful treatments (Young, 1997). If patients are losing weight or have severe vomiting, admission to hospital with the administration of intravenous fluids and an NG tube may be necessary, or even a gastrostomy tube.

(7) *Bladder dysfunction.* The bladder may be emptied by mechanical methods such as simple manual pressure or intermittent self-catheterization (Fox and Pickering, 1995). Long-term antibiotics may be necessary if recurrent urinary tract infections occur.

(8) *Respiratory/cardiac arrests.* Young (1997) emphasizes the need for meticulous cardiorespiratory monitoring during the perioperative period in patients with autonomic neuropathy.

Diabetic mononeuropathies

Single nerves are affected. Onset is rapid, recurrence is rare, symptoms are usually severe and patients recover. They are more common in men and in older patients but can develop at any age or duration of diabetes. Diabetic mononeuropathies include amyotrophy, cranial nerve palsies and truncal radiculopathies.

Amyotrophy is the most common and will therefore be discussed in this chapter.

Proximal motor neuropathy (amyotrophy)

This is characterized by pain with or without wasting of the thigh. It typically affects those over 50 years of age and may occur in Type 2 diabetes or Type 1 diabetes. The quadriceps may become wasted and weak, making walking up stairs difficult. One or both thighs may be affected at presentation (Watkins and Edmonds, 1997). Pain usually begins to decrease after three months and resolves after a year. Some wasting may remain but weakness is uncommon and recurrence unlikely. The cause of amyotrophy is unknown.

Diagnosis/symptoms

The patient finds it difficult to rise from a squatting position. The knee jerk is absent and the ankle jerk may be intact. Other causes of wasting of the quadriceps should be excluded.

Management

Some authorities believe that tight control improves the condition, particularly treatment with insulin (Fox and Pickering, 1995). Physiotherapy may be both physically and psychologically supportive (Young, 1997).

Pressure palsies/compressive mononeuropathies

Carpal tunnel syndrome is the most common compressive mononeuropathy occurring in people with diabetes. It involves the swelling of the median nerve which is then compressed by surrounding structures. This leads to the development of 'pins and needles' and sometimes numbness in the fingers, hand, wrist or forearm. Diagnosis is confirmed by nerve conduction studies. Treatment is by surgical decompression of the carpal tunnel.

Ulnar nerve compression at the elbow also occurs more commonly in those with diabetes. Management involves education of patients to avoid leaning on their elbow. The common peroneal nerve may be damaged at the neck of the fibula. This is rare and may lead to foot drop (Fox and Pickering, 1995).

Sexual Dysfunction in Men with Diabetes

Erectile failure is usually called impotence, although Fox and Pickering claim that this is politically incorrect. The term implies that because of the failure to achieve an erection a man loses all his power. Erectile failure is defined as the inability to achieve or sustain an erection sufficient for sexual intercourse.

Sexual dysfunction is a common problem in men with diabetes. According to Alexander (1997) 30 per cent of all men with diabetes and 55 per cent over 60 years old have erectile failure. This is likely to be an underestimate. Erectile dysfunction can cause distress to both patients and their partners.

Effects of diabetes

Diabetes can affect the erectile process in a number of ways.

Blood glucose control

Poor glycaemic control may lead to lethargy and loss of sexual interest. Balanitis due to candida infection may also occur in those with poorly controlled diabetes and may discourage intercourse.

Psychological factors

Fear of diabetic complications (including impotence), depression, anxiety and relationship difficulties may all lead to erectile failure.

Vascular disease

Atheroma of the arteries supplying the corpora or the pudendal arteries may lead to reduced blood flow. Involvement of the internal iliac arteries leads to Leriche syndrome with erectile failure and intermittent claudication in the thighs and buttocks. Failure of the veno-occlusive mechanism will lead to premature detumescence. Hypercholesterolaemia may induce corpus cavernosum fibrosis and the smooth muscle of the corpus itself may be damaged.

Neuropathy

Diabetic neuropathy can affect both erection and ejaculation. Fox and Pickering (1995) argue that autonomic neuropathy is the most common cause of impotence in men with diabetes.

Drugs

Some drugs which are commonly used by patients with diabetes may be implicated in erectile failure. These include (1) antihypertensives, in particular beta-blockers, thiazide diuretics and methyldopa; (2) antidysrhythmic drugs, e.g. verapamil; (3) lipid-lowering drugs, e.g. fibrates; (4) psychotropic drugs, e.g. antidepressants; (5) other drugs such as allopurinol, cimetidine, ketoconazole, metoclopramide and non-steroidal anti-inflammatory agents; (6) social drugs such as alcohol, cannabis and smoking (Alexander, 1997).

Endocrine disorders

These are less common causes of erectile dysfunction in men with diabetes.

Testicular failure and hyperprolactinaemia are causative. Allen (1998) claims that a primary physical cause can be identified in 97–98 per cent of cases.

The role of the nurse

It is not uncommon for the man with diabetes to talk to DSNs or practice nurses about sexual dysfunction. It is therefore vital for the nurse to be aware of the types of sexual problems which may occur, the likely causes and the investigations which may be required. He or she should also be able to describe the treatments available. Patient information material produced by Diabetes UK is available (at a cost) and Owen Mumford produces a leaflet written by Dr Alexander (free of charge), available by telephone via their Impotence Careline (Tel: 01993 812433). Diabetes centres should have leaflets available and easily accessible. There is also an impotence association:

The Impotence Association
PO Box 10296
London SW17 7ZN, UK
Tel: 020 8767 7791

In order to find out the cause of the problem, whether treatment is desired and which treatment is most suitable, a detailed history and examination are necessary. Where possible, and with the patient's agreement, the patient's partner should be present. It is important to find out from the patient and his partner how important the problem is to them. Allen (1998) claims that in her experience two-thirds of partners do not attend and she argues that this should not prevent treatment being offered.

Patients should be asked about libido. Reduced sexual interest may be due to anxiety, depression or problems with the relationship. Loss of libido may also be associated with other endocrine disorders such as hypogonadism. Does the patient have partial or complete erectile failure? Does he wake in the morning with an erection? Does premature ejaculation occur? Are there any painful conditions of the penis, such as thrush, or any change in the appearance of the penis, for example as in Peyronie's disease?

Questions regarding drug and alcohol intake or a history of bladder or bowel disorder or intermittent claudication may indicate a physical cause.

Psychological causes are more likely if early morning or nocturnal erections occur spontaneously; a patient may achieve erections sometimes with his partner or more particularly if away from the partner. If psychological in origin, the onset is likely to be sudden.

A full medical examination of the genitalia and the cardiovascular and peripheral nervous systems should be undertaken. Blood should be analysed for HbA1$_c$, creatinine, prolactin, testosterone and sex-hormone-binding globulin levels (Alexander, 1997).

A single cause may not be found. Treatment options such as vacuum devices and intracavernous injections may be effective regardless of the underlying cause. Psychological counselling can be beneficial to all, by encouraging communication and understanding between partners.

Treatment/management options

- improvement of glycaemic control
- replacing prescribed drugs which may cause erectile failure
- correcting any hormonal deficiencies (Allen, 1998 claims that creams and gels are usually ineffective)
- counselling – performed by a psychologist or psychiatrist if psychological factors are the primary cause
- intracorporeal injection of vasoactive agents such as papaverine or prostaglandin E. These can be self-injected by the patient into the corpus cavernosum. Potential side-effects include bruising, priapism (prolonged erection), fibrosis of injection sites and syncope. Patients can be educated about these risks and how they can be prevented. Satisfaction rates have been reported to be as high as 75 per cent (Sidi et al., 1988). Prescriptions for these drugs can be obtained free of charge, which may make this treatment more attractive to those on a low budget
- medicated urethral system for erection (MUSE). This involves the insertion of a pellet into the urethra and may be more acceptable to those with needle phobias (Allen, 1998). Like other prescription drugs, it is available free of charge to those with diabetes
- vacuum tumescence devices. These apply a vacuum when a rigid closed plastic tube is placed over the penis and a hand- or battery-operated pump is used. When erection occurs a rubber constriction ring is slipped over the tube on to the base of the penis to maintain erection. An understanding partner is required and the device is fairly tricky to use. Problems include a cool penis and the battery-operated pump is noisy. Devices cost in the range of £150 upwards and are available directly from the manufacturer, who provides education leaflets, videos and a helpline. Satisfaction rates are around 60–80 per cent (Fox and Pickering, 1995)
- oral Viagra (sildenafil) a phosphodiesterase-5-inhibitor which increases penile response to sexual stimulation. This has been given an extremely high profile in the media, and is available on prescription for men with diabetes. Viagra is contraindicated in patients taking nitrates. Although effective in patients with diabetes (57 per cent of Viagra-treated patients reported improved erections in a study by Rendell and Moreno, 1998) it is not as effective as in men without diabetes. Alexander (1998) argues that it may prove least effective in those with Type 2 diabetes and vascular disease and most successful for men whose problem is predominantly neuropathic. The main side-effects of Viagra are headache, flushing, diarrhoea, dyspepsia and visual disturbance. Priapism does not appear to be a problem. Obvious benefits over other treatments include its discreet and non-invasive administration method, and that it only works when the man is sexually stimulated and rarely causes priapism.

- congenital or other physical abnormalities may be corrected by surgery
- a semi-rigid rod may be inserted into the corpus cavernosum. In practice these are often reserved for men for whom other treatments have been ineffective.

Alexander (1997) found that in the centre in which he worked, 30 per cent of men did not want treatment after a full discussion of the problems and treatment options. Of those who wanted treatment, 70 per cent chose self-injection, the remainder a vacuum device. Allen (1998) reported that 78 per cent of her patients achieved satisfaction with vacuum devices.

Macrovascular Complications

Macrovascular complications refer to disease affecting the arteries that supply the heart, brain and legs, which may result in heart disease, stroke and peripheral vascular disease. Macrovascular disease is not exclusive to diabetes and causes high morbidity and mortality in the general population. The reduction of cardiovascular disease in all people by 30–40 per cent is a key Health of the Nation (Department of Health, 1992) target. It is suggested that this be achieved by reducing the prevalence of smoking, the intake of saturated fats, obesity and blood pressure levels and by an increase in exercise.

In most studies, Type 2 diabetes and Type 1 diabetes are examined together; here both Type 2 and Type 1 diabetes will be referred to as diabetes unless otherwise stated. The results will therefore apply mostly to Type 2 diabetes as this is the more common form of the disease.

Diabetes increases the risk of coronary heart disease by two to three times in men and four to five times in women (Fuller et al., 1980; Rosengren et al., 1989). The risk of stroke is increased two- to threefold (Bell, 1994). Women with diabetes lose their pre-menopausal protection from cardiovascular disease.

Diabetes is associated with socioeconomic factors. Prevalence of, and mortality associated with, diabetes is less in those from higher social groups (Yudkin et al., 1996). In those with diabetes, this pattern is reinforced. Diabetes is, however, an independent risk factor for cardiovascular disease. Yudkin et al. (1996) claim that 75–90 per cent of the excess risk of coronary artery disease in people with diabetes remains when adjusted for other known risk factors.

The prevalence of diabetes is substantially higher in South Asian and Afro-Caribbean people (see Chapter 6). There are greatly increased mortality risks of ischaemic heart disease among South Asian people with diabetes and of strokes in Afro-Caribbean people with diabetes.

McKeigue et al. (1991) argue that conventional risk factors such as smoking, cholesterol and hypertension cannot account for the high rates of coronary heart disease in South Asian people. They implicate insulin resistance and central obesity, which will be discussed later in this chapter.

The high levels of blood pressure in Afro-Caribbean patients with diabetes may account for the high rates of strokes and coronary artery disease when compared with Europeans.

Possible risk factors

Glycaemic control in those with established diabetes

There is as yet no prospective study which demonstrates that 'tight' blood glucose control reduces the risk of coronary heart disease. The DCCT Research Group (1993) investigated microvascular rather than macrovascular disease and the UKPDS (1998a) found that intensive blood glucose control substantially reduced the risk of some microvascular but not macrovascular disease.

Impaired glucose tolerance (IGT)

Those with IGT show an increased risk of cardiovascular disease. Gerstein and Yusuf (1996) claim that a continuous relationship exists between raised blood glucose levels and the risk of cardiovascular disease.

Hypertension

During the course of the UKPDS it was found that 40 per cent of men and over 50 per cent of women had hypertension. After 4.6 years follow-up it was found that the combined risks of Type 2 diabetes and hypertension were greater than for Type 2 diabetes alone. The risk of a cardiac-related death was 1.8 per cent in the normotensive group compared with 3.6 per cent in the hypertensive group. Mortality from stroke was 0.2 per cent and 0.9 per cent respectively.

Cholesterol

Total levels of cholesterol are similar in those with and without diabetes. There are, however, differences found in subclasses of cholesterol in those with Type 2 diabetes. These include low levels of protective high-density lipoprotein (HDL) and an increase in very-low-density lipoprotein (VLDL), which may increase the risk of arteriosclerosis (Yudkin et al., 1996). Those with Type 2 diabetes also tend to have high levels of triglycerides which may be associated with an increased risk of coronary heart disease.

Smoking

The risks of smoking in the general population are well documented. Fox and Pickering (1995) claim that meta-analysis has shown that stopping smoking is better than any other intervention in decreasing cardiovascular disease and prolongs the life of an average man with diabetes by three years.

Syndrome X

Reaven (1988) claimed that patients with syndrome X are at serious risk of cardiovascular disease. Syndrome X consists of:

- insulin resistance
- glucose intolerance
- hyperinsulinaemia
- increased VLDL triglyceride
- decreased HDL cholesterol
- hypertension.

This pattern of association is not complete in all patients and varies among different cultures (Marks, 1996). High VLDL and low HDL cholesterol are associated with central obesity and a waist–hip ratio of >1 (see p. 16) (Fox and Pickering, 1995).

Avoiding obesity and increasing physical activity were recommended by Reaven (1998) to minimize the risk factors for coronary heart disease of syndrome X. Campbell and Purcell (2001) argue that syndrome X should be more appropriately named the 'silent sextet' since other characteristics that increase the risk of cardiovascular disease have been identified.

The six principal features of the cardiac risk cluster seen with Type 2 diabetes are:

- Central obesity
- Glucose intolerance and Type 2 diabetes (insulin resistance and hyperinsulinaemia)
- Hypertension
- Dyslipidaemia (increased triglycerides, reduced high density lipoprotein-cholesterol)
- Pro-coagulant state
- Atherosclerosis (Campbell and Purcell, 2001).

Screening (based on Yudkin et al., 1996; this is also covered in Chapter 8)

As a minimum:

- measurement of blood pressure at least annually. Technique should be as suggested by the British Hypertension Society
- fasting lipid profiles should be measured every three years (this is in direct contrast with Diabetes UK recommendations in *What Diabetes Care to Expect*: they recommend that lipids should be checked yearly)
- at annual review patients should be questioned about smoking and encouraged to stop. Nicotine replacement therapy should be provided as necessary
- weight should be monitored at least yearly and patients should be involved in the setting of realistic targets for weight loss (if necessary) and seen by a state-registered dietitian.

Unfortunately, cardiovascular disease is often present at the diagnosis of Type 2 diabetes. The following section will discuss ways to reduce the risks of cardiovascular disease.

Reducing the risk of cardiovascular disease

The following recommendations are based on those made by Yudkin et al. (1996) for the Report of the Cardiovascular Group to the BDA (now Diabetes UK) on the Implementation of the St Vincent Declaration and the National Service Framework for Coronary Heart Disease (Department of Health, 2000).

Education

The provision of an education programme for all people with diabetes at diagnosis is recommended. This should be evaluated and revised at regular intervals. The programme should be tailored to the individual's needs, and take account of language and culture. The emphasis should be on lifestyle measures which may help to prevent heart disease, e.g. stopping smoking, low-fat, low-salt diets, weight loss, etc. Please see Chapter 2 for information about diet and Chapter 4 regarding education.

Control of blood pressure

The benefits of reduction in blood pressure have been clearly demonstrated in those with Type 1 diabetes and those with Type 2 diabetes. In Type 1 diabetes they have been shown to confer a renal rather than a cardiovascular benefit. The UKPDS (1998a) showed tight blood pressure control to have both microvascular and macrovascular benefits. Initially, non-pharmacological measures as described above should be used in the treatment of hypertension in those with Type 2 diabetes.

Drug treatment is recommended in any Type 2 diabetes with BP over 140/80 mmHg (UKPDS, 1998a). The Hypertension Optimal Treatment (HOT) Study (Hansson et al., 1998) provides evidence for a blood pressure target of 135/80 mmHg. In the near future this may fall to 130/80 mmHg. The choice of anti-hypertensive drugs and the various advantages and disadvantages of each are beyond the scope of this book. The UKPDS, however, found that ACE inhibitors confer no greater benefit than beta blockers and that many patients require more than one drug to achieve target BP control.

Reduction of lipids

People with diabetes should be treated as other patients with known vascular disease (e.g. post myocardial infarction). The aims are to keep LDL cholesterol < 3.5 mmol/L and HDL cholesterol > 1.0 with fasting triglyceride 2.0 mmol/L and a total cholesterol of 5.2 mmol/L or less. Initially dietary measures are recommended, such as reduction in total fat intake, replacement of saturated fats with monounsaturated and polyunsaturated fatty acids (see p. 21) and improving glycaemic control.

Weight loss in the overweight patient with Type 2 diabetes has been shown to reduce triglyceride and cholesterol levels and also to increase life expectancy.

Treatment of dyslipidaemia should first be to lower LDL cholesterol, secondly to raise HDL cholesterol and thirdly to lower triglycerides (Watts, 2000). Statins are indicated in those with raised LDL/total cholesterol and low HDL, and fibrates may be used to control high triglyceride low HDL profiles.

Aspirin

Aspirin therapy, 75–300 mg enteric-coated once daily, is recommended for all people with diabetes with any evidence of macrovascular disease such as angina, previous myocardial infarction, peripheral vascular disease or stroke. Diabetes UK (2001) have extended the recommendation for aspirin to those with dyslipidaemia, hypertension, BMI greater than 25, those from an Indo-Asian background, smokers, or those with retinopathy, unless contraindicated. The Antiplatelet Trialists Collaboration (1994) found that aspirin produced similar reductions in vascular events in high-risk diabetic patients (17 per cent) to people without diabetes (22 per cent).

Lifestyle changes

(1) *Stopping smoking:* Yudkin et al. (1996) recommend making nicotine replacement therapy widely available on prescription to people with diabetes.
(2) *Physical activity:* Inactivity is a major risk factor for coronary heart disease. Increased physical activity, diet changes and weight loss have been shown to decrease BP by 7 per cent, cholesterol by 4 per cent and triglyceride concentration by 8 per cent in those with Type 2 diabetes (Eriksson and Lindgarde, 1990).

Other treatments

Diabetes carries twice the risk of death following acute myocardial infarction (AMI) as that of non-diabetic patients. Several treatments can however improve this:

(1) Thrombolytic therapy (reduction of mortality of up to 42 per cent)
(2) Aspirin – 300 mg enteric-coated daily
(3) Tight glycaemic control.
   Tight glycaemic control was investigated by the DIGAMI study (Diabetes Mellitus, Insulin Glucose Infusion in Acute Myocardial Infarction). (Malmberg, 1997). The study was unable to determine whether the improved outcome of patients treated with insulin was due to good glycaemic control during the event or following discharge, or whether stopping sulphonlyureas was the most significant factor. However its findings suggest that patients suffering an AMI should have an insulin/glucose infusion on admission and subcutaneous insulin following discharge.
(4) Long-term treatment with betablockers
(5) Coronary artery bypass grafting.

Feet

Diabetic foot problems involve neuropathy, ischaemia and infection, which may lead to tissue breakdown and an increased risk of amputation. In the mainly neuropathic foot, sensory deficits and autonomic dysfunction occur but there is good circulation. The purely ischaemic foot is rare in people with diabetes (Edmonds et al., 1996). The more appropriate term is therefore the neuro-ischaemic foot where neuropathy and the absence of foot pulses coexist.

Box 3.8: The differential diagnosis of the neuropathic and ischaemic foot

Neuropathic	(Neuro)-ischaemic
Absent sensation	Normal or slightly reduced sensation
Warm	Cool
Colour: normal to pink (may have dry/ cracked skin)	Colour: pale to cyanosed
Usually painless (but can be very painful, particularly at night)	Pain at rest
Palpable pulses	Absent pulses
Callus (commonly under the head of the first metatarsal)	Absent callus
Knee/ankle jerk diminished or absent	Knee/ankle jerk present

Complications

Neuropathic ulcer (found on sole of the foot)	Ulceration on the margins of the foot
Charcot joint	Gangrene

Edmonds and Foster (2000) identify six stages of the diabetic foot.

(1) The normal foot – no risk factors
   Action:
   • Control of blood glucose, lipids, BP, smoking and decent shoes should be ensured.
(2) The high-risk foot – oedema, neuropathy, plantar callus, ischaemia, sensation, or deformity not accommodated in footwear.
   Action:

- Extra depth shoe should be provided in case of deformity, and felt padding to relieve plantar pressures; also education is vital so that patients/carers can recognize danger signs.

(3) The ulcerated foot – the pivotal state on the route to amputation.
   Action:
   - wound control with regular debridement of neuropathic ulcers
   - microbiological control with inspection of the foot, swabs and antibiotics
   - mechanical control: casts, insoles in shoes, special shoes, palpation of pulses, measurement of brachial pressure index and perhaps angiography/revascularization for an ulcerated ischaemic foot
   - metabolic control of blood glucose, blood pressure, lipids and smoking
   - education – patients need to know danger signs, how to inspect the ulcer and how to clean, dress, rest or use special shoes or casts.

(4) The cellulitic foot – infection has taken hold.
   Action:
   - swabs for laboratory analysis and appropriate prescription of systemic antibiotics

(5) The necrotic foot.
   Action:
   - necrotic toes on neuropathic foot could be amputated and most feet heal quickly
   - ischaemic patients may need a distal bypass and require wound care for the large leg wounds left after the graft is harvested and the bypass inserted.

(6) The foot that cannot be rescued – major amputation inevitable.
   Action:
   - rehabilitation of patient and return the other foot to an earlier stage of risk.

Infection can complicate ulceration in both the neuropathic and neuro-ischaemic foot.

Many patients newly diagnosed with Type 2 diabetes already have 'at-risk' feet. Early recognition of the at-risk foot and intensive treatment of foot complications in multidisciplinary foot clinics has reduced the need for amputation. Edmonds et al. (1996) demonstrated that the setting up of a specialist foot clinic which involved a chiropodist, a shoe fitter, a nurse, a physician and a surgeon, reduced amputations.

The extent and cost of the problem

Foot ulceration and infection are the most common cause of hospitalization for patients with diabetes. Neil et al. (1987) found that people with diabetes are 15 times more likely to undergo a lower extremity amputation than the general population.

The costs to the NHS, to patients and their carers is high. Marks (1996) claims that in 1985–6 amputations and the cost of fitting artificial limbs cost

£13.4 million a year in the UK. This did not include costs borne by social services or by the patients themselves.

Risk factors

- Risk factors for peripheral vascular disease (PVD) include smoking, hypertension and elevated cholesterol.
- Increasing duration of diabetes increases the risk of both neuropathy and PVD.
- Hyperglycaemia in those with Type 1 diabetes increases the incidence of neuropathy (DCCT, 1993; UKPDS, 1998a).
- The presence of neuropathy is a risk factor for ulcer formation. If the ability to experience pain is lost, damage is more likely to occur.
- Those with poor vision and poor dexterity may injure their feet if cutting their own nails and be unable to see colour changes or breaks in the skin.
- Absence of family/social support increases the risk of amputation (Reiber, 1993).

Screening

What Diabetes Care to Expect (Diabetes UK, 2001) states that patients should have their feet examined annually by a health professional experienced in the care of diabetes. Referral should be made to a State Registered Chiropodist or Podiatrist as required. Edmonds et al. (1996) argue that the patients 'at risk' should be identified at this screening. Patients at high risk should receive specific foot care education in addition to general education given at diagnosis. Close chiropodial/podiatrial supervision should be arranged.

The examination of the foot

Fox and Pickering (1995) argue that throughout the foot examination the health professional should explain what he or she is doing, what he or she is looking for and describe the implications of the findings to the patient. The examination then becomes an educational activity where management strategies can be agreed.

Management

Education

Patients newly diagnosed with diabetes (particularly Type 2 diabetes) are commonly very worried about amputation. Perhaps posters on bus shelters or billboards or experiences of friends and family have contributed to this. Their fears should be explored and preventive education begun.

Box 3.9: The examination of the foot

(1) Look at the foot
- Colour, shape and temperature should be observed (see Box 3.8)
- Deformities such as hallux valgus, overriding toes, Charcot joint or rocker-bottom deformity need special shoes
- Thickened or hardened toe nails need chiropody
- Look carefully for corns or calluses; these need chiropody
- Check between toes for evidence of fungal infection (athlete's foot)

(2) Examine peripheral blood supply
- Posterior tibial and dorsalis pedis pulses should be checked. If absent, doppler testing should be used

(3) Examine peripheral nerve supply
- Vibration perception should be assessed with a tuning fork or a biothesiometer applied to the hallux
- Light touch sensation can be examined using the Semmes-Weinstein nylon monofilament or cotton wool
- Thermal thresholds and pain sensation should be assessed.

(4) Look at footwear
- Ensure that shoes are sensible, well fitting and not causing abnormal pressure (see Box 3.10)
- Ensure that socks are not too constrictive and that seams are not too thick (which may lead to ulcers)
- Check for foreign bodies, e.g. stones, or protrusion of nails or staples which may lead to injury

---

The education of the patient with diabetes is the responsibility of all health professionals. Education should occur at diagnosis and be reviewed regularly. Additional, more intensive, education should be given to those with feet 'at risk'. The information given should include the risks of smoking, and encouragement and support should be given to stop. Footwear advice, routine foot care advice, the importance of screening and what to do if problems occur should all be discussed (see Chapter 4 for a discussion of footcare education).

It is important that education should be specially aimed at the individual. For example, a young person with no evidence of neuropathy or ischaemia does not need to wear plastic shoes on the beach.

There is evidence to support the idea that good foot care can prevent foot complications. A prospective study at Kings College Hospital (Edmonds et al., 1996) demonstrated that tight, ill-fitting shoes were the most frequent precipitating cause of foot ulcers. Results were confirmed when 83 per cent of those who continued to wear unsuitable shoes had a recurrence of ulcer(s) compared with 26 per cent of those wearing specially fitted shoes.

> **Box 3.10: The requirements for diabetic shoes**
>
> • Broad, rounded or square toes
> • Adequate depth
> • Soft upper leather across the toes
> • Low heels (high heels lead to excessive pressure on the forefoot and squeeze toes together)
> • Lace up, velcro or buckle straps to prevent movement within the shoe
> • Soft heels
> • Feet should be measured for fitting when purchased

Feet at risk

As discussed, those with feet at risk require regular chiropody/podiatry. Those with sensory neuropathy, clawing of the toes and some patients with neuro-ischaemic feet require ready-made diabetic shoes (Edmonds et al., 1996).

Development of foot lesions

Rapid access to the hospital (foot clinic if available) for diagnosis and treatment is necessary. According to Edmonds et al. (1996), the hospital foot clinic should comprise a named chiropodist, diabetologist and a nurse, with assistance from an orthotist (shoe fitter), vascular surgeon and interventional radiologist.

Ulcers

• Step 1 should determine whether the ulcer is predominantly caused by ischaemia or neuropathy (see Box 3.8).
• Step 2 should determine whether infection is present.

Neuropathic ulcers

Neuropathic ulcers occur in areas of pressure. Urgent chiropody is needed to remove callus. If healing is delayed a plaster cast may be needed with a window cut over the ulcer. This allows healing, prevents pressure and preserves mobility. Prophylactic orthopaedic surgery may be necessary to reduce pressure and prevent further ulceration.

If infection is suspected, oral or intravenous antibiotics are needed. Topical antibiotics have no place in the management of diabetic ulcers. A swab should be taken before antibiotics are initiated. Oral antibiotics usually used are amoxicillin, flucloxacillin (gram positive), metronidazole (anaerobes) and ceftazidime (gram negative) in combination, often for periods of weeks.

If deep-rooted infection is suspected, urgent admission to hospital is necessary for bed rest and intravenous antibiotics. Debridement by the podiatrist or surgeon and daily dressings and foot inspection are required. Oral antibiotics can be given once the infection begins to heal. X-rays are necessary to confirm osteomyelitis.

Ischaemic ulcers

These are usually painful. As in neuropathic ulcers, antibiotics are required if infection is present and referral to a vascular surgeon is then required. Angiography or doppler and/or Duplex ultrasound should be used to assess the vascular supply. Angioplasty or bypass surgery should be considered as appropriate. Surgical debridement of an ischaemic foot may be necessary and Edmonds et al. (1996) argue that this should not be delegated to junior staff.

Arthropathy – Charcot joint

Charcot changes occur in 0.5 per cent of diabetic patients (Purewal, 1996) and occur in neuropathic feet. The foot becomes painful, swollen and hot, often after a small injury. A destructive phase then follows, and blood-flow to the bone increases, leading to bone resorption and softening. This is followed by a characteristic deformity which carries a high risk of ulceration.

Treatment

Purewal (1996) recommends that, if presenting early, a strict policy of non-weight-bearing for 8–12 weeks should be adopted (bed rest or plaster cast). Care should be taken to mobilize gently after this period. If treated in the acute phase, chronic deformity may be prevented.

In the chronic phase, where severe deformity and bone fragmentation has already occurred, the aim is to stabilize the joint and avoid pressure which may lead to ulceration. Plaster casts may be necessary. Specially made shoes will be necessary. Research is ongoing about the use of pamidronate which may reduce bone loss. If ulcers are present, infection should be treated aggressively with broad-spectrum antibiotics and the ulcers should be regularly debrided.

Amputation

Edmonds et al. (1996) argue that the amputation of an ischaemic limb should be undertaken only if the possibility of a revascularization procedure has been excluded by the vascular service. Furthermore, they believe that the institution of a multidisciplinary foot care programme can realistically achieve the target of 50 per cent reduction in amputations included in the St Vincent Declaration.

A major amputation may be necessary for severe pain from extensive gangrene. Rehabilitation should be given by a multidisclipary team attached to a limb-fitting centre.

National Service Framework

The NSF standards relevant to this chapter are shown in Box 3.11.

Box 3.11: NSF standards

Standard 3: Empowering people with diabetes

(3)   All children, young people and adults with diabetes will receive a service which encourages partnership in decision-making, supports them in managing their diabetes and helps them to adopt and maintain a healthy lifestyle. This will be reflected in an agreed and shared care plan in an appropriate format and language. Where appropriate, parents and carers should be fully engaged in this process.

Standard 7: Management of diabetic emergencies

(7)   The NHS will develop, implement and monitor agreed protocols for rapid and effective treatment of diabetic emergencies by appropriately trained health care professionals. Protocols will include the management of acute complications and procedures to minimize the risk of recurrence.

Standards 10, 11 and 12: Detection and Management of long-term complications

(10) All young people and adults with diabetes will receive regular surveillance for the long-term complications of diabetes.
(11) The NHS will develop, implement and monitor agreed protocols and systems of care to ensure that all people who develop long-term complications of diabetes receive timely, appropriate and effective investigation and treatment to reduce their risk of disability and premature death.
(12) All people with diabetes, requiring multi-agency support will receive integrated health and social care.

Questions (one for each learning outcome)

(1) Mrs Martin, aged 66 years, arrives in accident and emergency. She is drowsy and her blood glucose is 50 mmol/L. She does not have a previous diagnosis of diabetes. She is accompanied by her husband.
   (a)   What questions do you think that you should ask Mr Martin to help to determine which type of acute complication of diabetes his wife has?
   (b)   What further investigations should be performed and what do you expect them to show?
   (c)   What emergency management will be necessary?
   (d)   What long-term treatment will be necessary?

(2) Katharine Allen is 21 years old and has had Type 1 diabetes for five years. She has been away at university for the last three years and has not attended for any screening, until today. She is keen to know how she can reduce her risks of long-term complications. What would you suggest?

(3) Mr Clough 'mentioned' at the end of an education session that he and his wife have been having 'a few difficulties' with sex. He wants to know if it is to do with his diabetes. How do you respond?

Suggested responses are to be found on pp. 251–3.

References

Alberti KGMM (1974) Diabetic ketoacidosis – aspects of management. In Ledingham JG (Ed) Tenth Advanced Medicine Symposium. Tunbridge Wells: Pitman Medical, pp 68–82.

Alexander WD (1997) Sexual function in diabetic men. In Pickup JC, Williams G (Eds) Textbook of Diabetes. 2nd edn. Oxford: Blackwell Science, pp 59.1–59.12.

Alexander W (1998) A double-blind, placebo-controlled, flexible dose-escalation study assessing the efficacy and safety of sildenafil (Viagra). Diabetes Update Autumn: 18–19, 22.

Allen P (1998) Erectile dysfunction: a nurse led service. 1998 Oxford Symposium on Diabetes Care Lecture, 8 April.

American Diabetes Association (1993) Summary of Diabetes Control and Complications Trial, pp 1–5.

Antiplatelet Trialists Collaboration (1994) Collaborative overview of randomised trials of anti-platelet therapy 1: Prevention of death, myocardial infarction and stroke by prolonged antiplatelet therapy in various categories of patients. British Medical Journal 308: 81–106.

Bell DSH (1994) Stroke in the diabetic patient. Diabetes Care 17: 213–19.

British Diabetic Association (1993) The Diabetes Control and Complications Trial Reports Back. Balance August/September: 20.

Bruce J, McKennell A, Walker E (1991) Blind and partial sighted adults in Britain. The RNIB Survey 1991. London: HMSO .

Campbell IW (1999) UKPDS: Implications for management of Type 2 diabetes in the millennium. Practical Diabetes International. September 16 (6): 161–2.

Campbell IW, Purcell H (2001) The silent sextet. Editorial, The British Journal of Diabetes and Vascular Disease, August, 1(1): 3–6.

Clarke CM, Lee DA (1995) Prevention and treatment of the complications of diabetes. New England Journal of Medicine 332 (18): 1210–17.

DECODE Study Group (1999) Glucose tolerance and mortality: comparison of WHO and American Diabetes Association diagnostic criteria. The DECODE Study Group (Diabetes Epidemiology: collaborative analysis of diagnostic criteria in Europe). Lancet 354: 617–21.

Department of Health (1992) The Health of the Nation: A Strategy for Health in England. Cm 1986. London: HMSO.

Department of Health (2000) National Service Framework for Coronary Heart Disease. London: The Stationery Office.

Department of Health (2003) National Service Framework for Diabetes Delivery Strategy. London: HMSO.

De Vegt F, Dekker Jm, Ruhe MG, Stenhouwer CD, Nijpels G, Bouter LM, Heine RJ (1999) Hyperglycaemia is associated with all cause and cardiovascular mortality in the Hoorn population: The Hoorn Study. Diabetologia 42 (8): 928–31.

Diabetes Control and Complications Trial Research Group (1993) The effect of intensive treatment of diabetes on the development and progression of long-term complications in insulin-dependent diabetes mellitus. New England Journal of Medicine 329: 977–86.

Diabetes UK (2001) What Diabetes Care to Expect. London: Diabetes UK.

Donahue RP, Abbott RD, Reed DM, Yan OK (1987) Postchallenge glucose concentration and coronary heart disease in men of Japanese ancestry. Honolulu Heart Programme. Diabetes 36: 689–92.

Edmonds M, Foster AVM (2000) The future of diabetic foot care. Modern management and recent advances. Practical Diabetes International June 17 (4): 51–6.

Edmonds M, Boulton A, Buckenham N, Every N, Foster A, Freeman D, Gadsby R, Gibby O, Knowles A, Pooke M, Tovey F, Wolfe UJ (1996) Report of the Diabetic Foot and Amputation Group. Diabetic Medicine 13: S27–S42.

Eriksson KF, Lindgarde F (1990) Prevention of Type 2 (non insulin dependent) diabetes mellitus by diet and physical exercise: the 6 year Malmo Feasibility Study. Diabetologia 34: 891–8.

Ewing DJ, Clarke BF (1986) Diabetic autonomic retinopathy: present insights and future prospects. Diabetes Care 9: 648–65.

Ewing DJ, Campbell IW, Clarke BF (1980) The natural history of diabetic autonomic neuropathy. Quarterly Journal of Medicine 193: 95–108 .

Foster AVM, Eaton C, McConville DO, Edmonds ME (1994) Appplication of Opsite film: a new and effective treatment of painful diabetic neuropathy. Diabetic Medicine 11: 768–72.

Fox C, Pickering A (1995) Diabetes in the Real World. London: Class Publishing.

Fraser RJ, Horowitz M, Maddox AF, Harding PE, Chatterto BE, Dent J (1990) Hyperglycaemia slows gastric emptying in Type 1 (insulin dependent) diabetes mellitus. Diabetologia 33: 675–80.

Fuller JH, Shipley MJ, Rose G, Jarrett J, Keen M (1980) Coronary heart disease risk and impaired glucose tolerance: The Whitehall Study. Lancet I: 1373–6.

Gale EAM, Dornan L, Tattersall RB (1981) Severely uncontrolled diabetes in the over-fifties. Diabetologia 21: 25–8 .

Gallichan M (1999) The UKPDS: a diabetes nursing perspective. Journal of Diabetes Nursing 3(1): 8–12.

Gerstein HC, Yusuf S (1996) Dysglycaemia and risk of cardiovasular disease. Lancet 347: 949–50.

Grenfell A (1997) Clinical management of diabetic nephropathy. In Pickup JC, Williams G (Eds) Textbook of Diabetes. 2nd edn. Oxford: Blackwell Science, pp 54.1–54.19.

Grey RHB, Burns-Cox CJ, Hughes A (1989) Blind and partial sighted registration in Avon. British Journal of Ophthalmology 73: 88.

Guy RJC, Clarke CA, Malcolm PN, Watkins PJ (1985) Evaluation of thermal and vibration sensation in diabetic neuropathy. Diabetologia 28: 131–7.

Hansson L et al. (1998) The Hypertension Optimal Treatment (HOT) Study. 24 month data on blood pressure and tolerability. Lancet 351: 1755–62.

Herman WH, Crofford OB (1997) The relationship between diabetic control and complications. In Pickup JC, Williams G (Eds) Textbook of Diabetes. 2nd edn. Oxford: Blackwell Science.

Herman WH et al. (1983) An approach to the prevention of blindness in diabetes. Diabetes Care 6(6): 608–13.

Hurel S, Orr A, Arthur M, Swainston M, Kelly WF (1997) Diabetic ketoacidosis: diabetes education and health beliefs. Practical Diabetes International January/February 14(1): 9–11.

Jones D, Dolben J, Owens DR, Vora JP, Young S, Creagh FM (1988) Non-mydriatic polaroid photography in screening for diabetic retinopathy: evaluation in a clinical setting. British Medical Journal 1988 296: 1029.

Kelly WF et al. (1993) Influence of social deprivation on illness in diabetic patients. British Medical Journal 307: 1115–16.

Klein R, Klein BEK, Moss SE, Davis MD, Dernets DL (1988) Glycosylated haemoglobin predicts the incidence and progression of diabetic retinopathy. Journal of the American Medical Association 260: 2864.

Klein R, Klein BEK, Moss SE, Davis MD, Dernets DL (1984b) The Wisconsin Epidemiological Study of diabetic retinopathy 11: prevalence and risk of diabetic retinopathy when age at diagnosis is 30 years or more. Archives of Ophthalmology 102: 527.

Kohner E, Allwinkle J, Andrews R, Baker R, Brown F, Cheng H, Gray M, Grindey S, Koppei I, Martin B, Reckless J, Rothman D, Sculpher M, Talbot R, Vaughan N, Wilkinson J (1996) Report of the Visual Handicap Group. Diabetic Medicine 13(suppl. 4): s13–s26.

Krentz A, Nattress M (1997) Acute metabolic complications of diabetes: diabetic ketoacidosis, hyperosmolar non-ketotic syndrome and lactic acidosis. In Pickup JC, Williams G (Eds) Textbook of Diabetes. 2nd edn. Oxford: Blackwell Science, pp 39.1–39.23.

Lewis EJ, Hunsicker LG, Bain RP, Rhode RD for the Collaborative Study Group (1993) The effect of angiotensin-converting enzyme inhibition on diabetic nephropathy. New England Journal of Medicine 329: 1456–62.

Lewis MJ, Ferguson SC, Campbell IW, Nowroz IM (1996) A very unusual case of hyperosmolar coma. Practical Diabetes International 13(6): 195–7.

Lowe LP, Lin K, Greenland P, Metzger BE, Dyer AR, Stanler J (1997) Diabetes: an asymptomatic hyperglycaemia and 22 year mortality in black and white men. The Chicago Heart Association Detection Projects in Industry Study. Diabetes Care 20: 163–9.

MacCuish AC (1992) Who should screen for diabetic retinopathy? Diabetes Reviews 1(1): 5–8.

Malmberg K (DIGAMI Study Group) (1997) Prospective randomised study of intensive insulin treatment on long-term survival after acute myocardial infarction. British Medical Journal 314: 1512–5.

Marks L (1996) Counting the Cost: The Real Impact of Non-Insulin Dependent Diabetes. London: Kings Fund Policy Institute/BDA.

McKeigue PM, Shah B, Marmott MG (1991) relation of central obesity and insulin resistance with high diabetes prevalence and cardiovascular risk in South Asians. Lancet 337: 382–6.

Microalbuminuria Collaborative Study Group UK (1995) Intensive therapy and progression to clinical albuminuria in patients with insulin dependent diabetes mellitus and microaluminuria. British Medical Journal 311: 973–7.

Nathan DM (1993) Long-term complications of diabetes mellitus. New England Journal of Medicine 328(23): 1676–85.

Nathan DM, Fogel HA, Godine JE et al. (1991) Role of diabetologist in evaluating diabetic retinopathy. Diabetes Care 14: 26–33.

National Screening Committee (2000) Preservation of Sight in Diabetes in England. http://www.neth.nhs.uk/screening/diabetic retinopathy.

Neil HAW, Gatling W, Mather HM, Thompson AV, Thorogood M, Fowler GH, Hill RD, Mann JL (1987) The Oxford Community Diabetes Study: evidence for an increase in the prevalence of known diabetes in Great Britain. Diabetic Medicine 4: 539–43.

O'Hare JP, Hopper A, Madhaven C, Charny M, Purewal TS, Harney B, Griffiths J (1996) Adding retinal photography to screening for diabetic retinopathy: a prospective study in primary care. British Medical Journal 312: 679-82.

Pirart J (1978) Diabetes mellitus and its degenerative complications: a prospective study of 4,400 patients observed between 1947 and 1973. Diabetes Care 1: 168–88.

Purewal TS (1996) Charcot's diabetic neuroarthropathy: pathogenesis, diagnosis and management. Practical Diabetes International 13(3) 88–9.

Reaven GM (1988) The role of insulin resistance in human disease. Diabetes 37: 1595–1607.

Reiber GE (1993) Epidemiology of the diabetic foot. In Levin ME, O'Neal W, Bowker JH (Eds) The diabetic Foot. 5th edn. St Louis: Mosby Year Book, pp 1–5.

Rendell M, Moreno F (1998) Viagra. Diabetes 47 (Suppl.): A90033.

Rohan TE, Frost CD, Wald NJ (1989) Prevention of blindness by screening for retinopathy: a quantitative assessment. British Medical Journal 299: 1198.

Rosengren A, Welin L, Tsioglanni et al. (1989) Impact of cardiovascular risk factors on coronary heart disease and mortality among middle aged diabetic men: a general population study. British Medical Journal 299: 1127–31.

Sidi AA, Reddy PA, Chen KK (1988) Patient acceptance of and satisfaction with vasoactive intracavernosal pharmacotherapy for impotence. Journal of Urology 140: 293–4.

Steno Study Group (1982) Effect of 6 months of strict metabolic control on eye and kidney function in insulin dependent diabetics with background retinopathy. Lancet 1: 121.

Stout RW (1991) Diabetes mellitus and old age. In Pickup J, Williams G (Eds) Textbook of Diabetes. Oxford: Blackwell Scientific, pp 897–904.

Trevison R, Barnes D, Viberti G (1997) The pathogenesis of diabetic nephropathy. In Pickup JC, Williams G (Eds) Textbook of Diabetes. 2nd edn. Oxford: Blackwell Science.

UK Prospective Diabetes Study Group (1998a) Intensive blood-glucose control with sulphonylureas or insulin compared with conventional treatment and risk of complications in patients with Type 2 diabetes (UKPDS 33) Lancet 352: 837–53.

UK Prospective Diabetes Study Group (1998b) Tight blood pressure control and risk of macrovascular and microvascular complications in Type 2 diabetes (UKPDS 39) British Medical Journal 317: 713–20.

UK Prospective Diabetes Study Group (1998c) Effect of intensive blood-glucose control with metformin on complications in overweight patients with Type 2 diabetes (UKPDS 34) Lancet 352: 854–65.

UK Prospective Diabetes Study Group (1998d) Cost effectiveness analysis of improved blood pressure control in hypertensive patients with Type 2 diabetes (UKPDS 40) British Medical Journal 317: 720–6.

UK Prospective Diabetes Study Group (2000) Cost effectiveness of an intensive blood glucose policy in patients with Type 2 diabetes: economic analysis alongside randomized controlled trial (UKPDS 41) British Medical Journal 320: 1373–8.

Valez R, Haffner S, Stern MP, von Hewison WAJ (1987) Ophthalmologist vs retinal photographs in screening for diabetic retinopathy. Clinical Research 35: 363.

Viberti GC, Morgenson CE, Groop LC, Pauls JF – The European Microalbuminuria Captopril Study Group (1994) Effect of captopril on progression to clinical proteinuria in patients with insulin-dependent diabetes mellitus and microalbuminuria. Journal of the American Medical Association 274: 275–9.

Viberti, GC, Marshall S, Beech R, Brown V, Derben P, Higson N, Home P, Keen H, Plant M, Walls J (1996) Report on renal disease in diabetes. Diabetic Medicine 13 (Suppl 4): S6–S12.

Walker JD, Bending JS, Dodds RA, Mattock MB, Murrells TJ, Keen H (1989) Restriction of dietary protein and progression of renal failure in diabetic nephropathy. Lancet 2: 1411–15.

Ward JD, Tesfaye S (1997) Pathogenesis of diabetic retinopathy. In Pickup JC, Williams G (Eds) Textbook of Diabetes. 2nd edn. Oxford: Blackwell Science, pp. 49.1–49.19.

Warshaw AL, Feller ER, Lee KH (1977) On the cause of raised serum amylase in diabetic ketoacidosis. Lancet 1: 929–31.

Watkins PJ, Edmonds ME (1997) Clinical features of diabetic retinopathy. In Pickup JC, Williams G (Eds) Textbook of Diabetes. 2nd edn. Oxford: Blackwell Science, pp. 50.1-50.20.

Watts GF (2000) Coronary disease, dyslipidaemia and clinical trials in Type 2 diabetes mellitus. Practical Diabetes Int. 17(2): 54–9.

Young R (1997) Management of neuropathy in Pickup JC, Williams G (Eds) Textbook of Diabetes. 2nd edn. Oxford: Blackwell Science, pp. 51.1–15.13

Young RJ, Ewing DJ, Clarke BF (1988) Chronic and remitting painful diabetic polyneuropathy: correlations with presenting clinical features and subsequent changes in neurophysiology. Diabetes Care 11: 34–40.

Yudkin JS, Blauth C, Drury PL, Fuller J, Henley T, Lancaster J, Lankester M, Lean M, Pentecost B, Press V, Rothman D (1996) Prevention and management of cardiovascular disease in patients with diabetes mellitus: an evidence base. Diabetic Medicine 13: S101–S121.

SECTION TWO
PATIENT EDUCATION AND CLINICAL MANAGEMENT OF DIABETES

Chapter 4
The education of the person with diabetes

This chapter addresses the learning needs of those with diabetes. It is divided into three sections: (1) the general principles of education; (2) the education of those with Type 1 diabetes; and (3) the education of those with Type 2 diabetes.

The information that the health care professional feels the patient needs and the information that the patient knows he or she needs may differ. Needs also vary between individuals and at different stages of life. Methods used to give information should differ according to individual preferences; for example, some may prefer group, others individual, education. The amount of time available, the availability of suitable literature, the environment and communication skills may all influence the success of diabetes education.

Learning Outcomes

After reading this chapter you should be able to:

(1) demonstrate an understanding of how diabetes education should be approached;
(2) provide basic education for those with Type 1 diabetes;
(3) undertake diabetes education for those with Type 2 diabetes.

Section One: The Principles of Education

Why educate?

Logic would imply that those with the greatest knowledge about diabetes and its management would have the best control of their blood glucose levels. Lockington et al. (1988) concluded that poor knowledge does prevent good control but that good knowledge does not automatically ensure good control. Attitudes rather than knowledge were found to be more strongly related to blood glucose control. Day (1996) claims that many psychosocial factors have shown stronger relationships with favourable behavioural outcomes than has education. These include health beliefs such as the severity of, or vulnerability to, short- and long-term complications; the locus of control, i.e. with whom the responsibility for care of diabetes lies, the social environment in which people operate and their general emotions. Psychological factors are discussed in more detail in Chapter 7. Educators need to take psychosocial factors into account and start at where the patient is.

Jervell (1996) claims that education can prevent over 70 per cent of episodes of diabetic ketoacidosis. It is clear that the skills and knowledge imparted must vary to satisfy diverse needs. The World Health Organisation (WHO) (1984) argues that health promotion (of which education is a part) should be the process of enabling people to increase control over and improve their health. Diabetes education should therefore allow patients to make informed decisions about their lifestyles and their diabetes care. The information given should be based on what the individual needs to make informed decisions.

Difficulties and considerations

Encouraging patients to make informed decisions about their health and 'allowing' them to make their own mistakes may be difficult for health care professionals. Delaney (1991) claims that health workers have difficulty accepting patients' rights not to conform. They argue that although empowerment and choice are acknowledged to contribute to health and well-being, we continue to seek 'compliance' and they beg the question of whether this promotes or impairs health.

The Black Report and The Health Divide (Townsend et al., 1992) identified marked inequalities in health status between social classes, in favour of the higher classes at all ages and in both sexes. Inequalities also existed in the utilization of health services ascribable to a complex under-provision in working-class areas and a perception of high financial and psychological cost versus perceived benefits. Whether socioeconomic differences are measured by occupational class, housing tenure, income, car ownership, economic status or education, differences occur and have been found in studies using many methods (Fox and Benzeval, 1995). Similarly, health inequalities exist in ethnic minority groups.

Blaxter (1983) claims that health-damaging behaviour may be inevitable in certain environments. Graham (1993) found that smoking was chosen as a coping strategy by working-class women. Education regarding healthy eating or smoking may therefore face more barriers in an area with a high working-class population.

The health beliefs of patients influence how much effect education will have. If a patient has a fatalistic view of life, lifestyle changes will not be seen as likely to affect outcome and are therefore unlikely to be made. Education needs to focus on these beliefs; a list of dos and don'ts will not suffice. Health beliefs are discussed more fully on pages 200–1.

Barriers to change need to be identified. The most important influence on the patient's life may actually be opposed to the advice given by health workers. A patient may believe that giving up smoking will lead to weight gain, a disaster if the patient is a model. Self-efficacy is important to achieve change; individuals need to believe that they can achieve the goal. Realistic achievable goals should be set, agreed and reviewed. A positive approach should be used to increase self-esteem.

What errors do we need to avoid?

Shillitoe (1992), a psychologist who has Type 1 diabetes, suggested how not to educate those with diabetes based on his own unfortunate experiences of health education.

Box 4.1: How not to educate (based on Shillitoe, 1992)

(1) Never give practical demonstrations. Explain rather than demonstrate practical skills such as blood testing (particularly ineffective if English is not the first language!)

(2) Always give unnecessary choices. If one method of injection works for a patient why not encourage them to try another?

(3) Use jargon – avoid short words

(4) Make yourself as inaccessible as possible. Never give your telephone number and ensure that you never see a patient more than once

(5) Think long term. Particularly ineffective in younger people who prefer short-term goals

(6) What's good for one is good for all. Use negative comparisons with others, e.g. Jim copes with his injections and he only has one arm

(7) Always blame the patient. Resist any temptation to wonder whether the treatment regime is appropriate or whether you have explained things clearly

(8) Take every opportunity to contradict both your colleagues and yourself

(9) Be vague not specific. Don't allow patients to ask questions, this could reduce confusion

(10) Stifle initiative. Remember, just because patients know themselves and what works best for them better than you do, you are the professional

---

How should we educate?

Acknowledge the irony inherent in the tips in Box 4.1. I would add that we need to listen to the patient before giving any information or advice.

Coles (1989) sees learning as linking information. He describes contextual learning theory and sees the role of the health care professional as less one of information-giving and more one of context-setting and relating the information to the understanding of the individual. He argues that education should be based on making connections and uses the analogy of a jigsaw puzzle. The first stage involves identifying the context of learning (the picture on the box); the second, making available appropriate information (the pieces inside the box);

the third, allowing learners actively to handle information for themselves and relate it to their own situation (fitting together the pieces to make the picture). He likens the role of the educator to that of the parent.

Before embarking on information-giving it is important to find out what the person already knows about diabetes. Ask what he or she would like to know, does he or she have any questions? Are there any problems which he or she is experiencing? It is also important that shared short-term achievable goals are negotiated. Day (1996) found that many patients set glycaemic goals which differed from those of health care professionals. He found that there were also wide variations set between professionals. It is important that information given by professionals is consistent, accurate and complete. Kaplan et al. (1985) found that the less controlling the professional the more the patient learnt and the better the $HbA1_c$ result. They also found that the higher the emotional content, the better the outcome. Day (1996) argues that from studies using video and audio tapes of interviews this is not often achieved. The agenda is often controlled by the professional and relates only to the medical aspects of the condition. Day (1996) argues that this is likely to be inappropriate.

In a 'nutshell' patients should be treated as individuals and education programmes planned according to their needs. Professionals should begin by evaluating the knowledge that the patient already has and by discussing any fears or concerns which may be barriers to learning. Time should be allowed for people to ask questions and these should be taken seriously. Understanding should be checked regularly before additional information is given. Achievable goals should be set and agreed with patients. Finally, information should be given in small, easily manageable pieces, and knowledge which the patient already has should be built upon. People with diabetes want information to help them solve problems which their individual daily life with diabetes presents.

People learn in different ways and at different paces. Some may be able to read and write English; some may be illiterate; some may be able to read another language; others may have visual problems that make reading difficult and may just prefer other ways of saving information. It is important to provide varied and interesting ways to give and reinforce information and also to provide a way for patients to continue to be updated. Diabetes UK provide various publications (some free) and they also have a website (www.diabetes.org.uk) which contains up-to-date information. The majority of Diabetes UK information continues to be in English although some leaflets are available in Asian languages. Many pharmaceutical companies provide 'free' education literature and videos for patients and some provide videos for Asian people with diabetes which are available in a variety of languages.

A computer-assisted learning package has been designed by the Ipswich Diabetes Centre, which allows patients to pick out information as required and learn at their own pace. Although expensive (approx. £200) it can be used within the diabetes centre, thus benefitting many patients, or lent to patients for use at home. It encourages active learning by asking questions and allowing patient responses, and giving information as required.

Wiley (publishers) have a diabetes website for those living and working with diabetes: www.diabetesonestop.com, and Abbott/Medisense also have a website: www.diabetesnow.co.uk. Both these sites are free to register with.

Use of checklists

Many professionals use education checklists. These can be useful for documenting information and I personally found them very useful as a memory jolt when I was a new DSN. However, they have limitations. Checklists are not specific to the individual and assume that people with the same disease need the same information. This may be true to some extent but individuals often need to know things in a different order, in varying amounts of detail, to have the information presented in different ways, and repetition may be required in different areas. Individual questions will also need to be addressed before the information is given. Walker (1993) gives three reasons why caution is required if lists are to be used:

(1) Checklists are the professionals' idea of what information should be given; this may not concord with the information required by the person at his or her particular stage of diabetes.
(2) Completion of checklists rarely involves the patient. The professional decides when to cover the topic and ticks or signs against the subject when they deem fit.
(3) There is a danger once a point on the list has been ticked, signed or dated that the professional will assume that it has been learnt. Education should be a continuous process rather than a one-off session with a checklist.

Group education

Group education sessions are commonly used and have a number of advantages. They are a cost-effective use of professional time (DSNs and dietitians are expensive resources). Patients who have diabetes are the real experts about living with the disease and their experiences and expertise can be drawn on during the sessions. Many patients have commented on how helpful it is to meet others with diabetes and so to feel that they are not alone. Setting aside a day, two mornings or a few evenings for education helps to give the message that education and patient experiences are important. If the number of people with diabetes and their partners or friends outnumber professionals in the group, this may help patients to feel more confident and empowered. The relaxed atmosphere usually helps too.

Perhaps the greatest strength of groups can be the interaction between members. Previously unspoken fears are often shared. For example, one man admitted his fear of blood testing; other group members acknowledged this fear and gave support and advice on how this could be overcome. In another group a woman admitted that she had been frightened to eat bananas for three years; the next morning other group members brought in bananas to share.

There are, however, disadvantages and potential problems in using groups. Facilitation of the group demands a high level of skill from the professional. This is particularly true when the session is unstructured or semi-structured (the best are) and allows patients to ask questions and cover topics in the order that they wish. The professional needs an excellent knowledge of diabetes in addition to good communication and management skills. Some patients may not contribute; the facilitator needs to ensure that they are included by asking them open questions which they are confident to answer. One person may monopolize the discussion, excluding other members. It requires skill to include this patient's ideas, stop him or her from talking without causing offence and include other group members. If a patient is pessimistic or has established complications of diabetes, others may become frightened or fatalistic and therefore reluctant to make lifestyle changes.

Planning of group sessions is essential. The group should be no more than 8–12 people and be in a relaxed informal environment. The chairs should be in a circle or semi-circle (not rows) and tea and coffee should be available. It is helpful to ensure that people invited can hear well and can speak English. We make extensive use of question-and-answer techniques, use a video, food models and a quiz to provide variety and to facilitate both active and passive learning.

Group education for those converting to insulin from tablet treatment

Groups have traditionally been used for people with Type 2 diabetes or those with established Type 1 diabetes who are already on insulin. More recently group education sessions for patients converting to insulin have been used in the centre in which I work. Almond (Almond et al., 2001) has described her experiences of using such sessions to convert Type 2 diabetes patients to insulin. Thirty-three people were divided into six groups of four to six people, and each group had between five and seven 2-hour sessions over a 4–12 month period. Blood glucose results were openly discussed by the groups and patients gave ideas for improving control. There was a mean reduction in HbA1$_c$ of 2.6 per cent and minimal weight gain. The groups were patient led and perceived as fun and confidence boosting. Importantly, in view of the projected increase in diabetes, there was a 25 per cent saving in professional time with the groups.

Models for education of people with diabetes

NICE (the National Institute for Clinical Excellence) will be appraising patient education models for diabetes in 2003. One model that is likely to be examined is DAFNE (the Dose Adjustment For Normal Eating education programme). This project, which has been shown to be successful in terms of reduced blood glucose levels and improved quality of life (particularly with regard to dietary freedom) in Germany, is currently undergoing trials in four centres in the UK.

The DAFNE programme educates people with Type 1 diabetes on how to adjust their insulin to fit in with their lifestyle. It involves a group 5-day outpatient training course in which 'DAFNE-trained' DSNs and dietitians provide the key input (Heller, 2001).

The Department of Health's Expert Patients Programme (DoH, 2001a) (currently being piloted in primary care) offers opportunity for people living with chronic disease to learn new skills to manage their condition. More information can be found on www.ohn.gov.uk/ohn/people/expert.htm

The Organization of Sections Two and Three

For ease of reference I have divided the next sections so as to indicate the broad educational needs of those with Type 2 diabetes and those with Type 1 diabetes. I have chosen to introduce the education of those with Type 1 diabetes in Section 2, taking a day-by-day approach beginning on the day of diagnosis. Section 3, which addresses the education of those with Type 2 diabetes, does not conform to a time scale.

Obviously, individual needs and priorities will differ. These sections should not be used as a formula applicable to every patient, merely as a guide to the process of educating people with diabetes. Topics need to be returned to, revised, and additional information given. In practice I use opportunistic methods and discuss subjects such as sick-day rules as opportunities present themselves.

Balance for Beginners – magazine-style education booklets – are available from Diabetes UK (formerly the British Diabetic Association) for those with Type 1 diabetes and those with Type 2 diabetes. These are excellent, although expensive for magazines.

Section Two: The Education of Those with Newly Diagnosed Type 1 Diabetes

Those who have just been diagnosed as having Type 1 diabetes are often frightened and apprehensive. The diagnosis may give rise to a diversity of emotions and people need to try to make sense of what has happened. Reactions may vary from relief – for example 'Thank goodness that I haven't got cancer'; 'At least there is an explanation and I will feel better' – to terror about injections, complications and having an incurable disease. Parents may feel guilty that they have given their child diabetes and patients may search for past events or behaviour which has made them deserve diabetes. Others may stand to lose their job.

In the midst of this emotion, people need to learn how to manage the physical side of diabetes. These physical needs tend to dominate initially, i.e. insulin injections. However, many patients feel that coming to terms with their feelings is as hard or even harder than learning about the diet, tests and injections. Emotional support and reassurance are therefore necessary.

How should we start?

I intend to take a day-by-day approach.

Day 1

Privacy is important; there should be no interruptions. Always start by asking if your patient has any previous experience of diabetes. Someone may have either positive or negative experiences. For example, a family member who copes well with diabetes, a Spurs supporter who knows of Gary Mabbutt's achievements, or very negative experiences: 'my mother died from renal failure'; 'I've seen those adverts on the bus shelter – gangrene, blindness and injections'. These issues should be addressed first.

An explanation

A clear simple explanation should be given. Explain the symptoms of which he or she complains, why he or she feels thirsty, passes lots of urine, feels tired, etc. and why insulin injections are necessary (see p. 4). An anatomy and physiology lesson is not helpful; it is not an opportunity for the nurse or doctor to demonstrate how clever they are. The patient should be reassured that the symptoms will quickly disappear. It is important to be honest and tell patients that there is no cure for diabetes and that although it can be controlled, insulin injections will be necessary for life. Many will ask why they cannot be treated with tablets; a simple explanation of the difference between Type 1 diabetes and Type 2 diabetes may therefore be necessary, and that oral insulin is destroyed by stomach enzymes, making injections necessary.

Injections

The first injection needs to be got over as quickly as possible; until it is, patients will find it difficult to absorb any other information. The nurse should demonstrate on her or himself first with an empty syringe or pen. Then the nurse should draw up the insulin for the patient but ask him or her to inject him or herself. Perhaps suggest that the patient uses either the thigh or abdomen in which to inject initially (see Figure 4.1). These areas are easy to see, and allow the use of both hands. Insulin injections are usually painless and patients often breathe a sigh of relief when the injection is over.

It is important to adjust the technique if a pen is used. With a syringe, as soon as the plunger is depressed fully the injection of fluid ceases, but with a pen fluid may continue to be expelled through the needle after the plunger has been depressed. Annersten and Frid (2000) recommend that patients using a pen should be taught to hold the needle in for at least 20 seconds after depressing the plunger since clinically significant leakage of fluid occurs after 7 seconds.

Drawing up

The whole process of drawing up should be demonstrated and then broken down into stages. The patient should be given lots of opportunity to practise. It is important to make the process as simple as possible. Hyperglycaemia often causes blurred vision and for this reason we tend to use either 0.5 ml syringes and doses in increments of 5 units which are clearer to see, or pen devices. Only one type of insulin should be used; mixing (if appropriate) can be introduced in a couple of days when the patient is more confident (see Chapter 2 for a discussion of insulin therapy). Printed information with pictures should also be given; this is available from pharmaceutical companies free of charge.

Injection sites

Insulin should be injected at a 90° angle into the fat below the skin. The skin should be pinched up using the thumb and index finger/middle finger to ensure that insulin is not injected into muscle. Swabbing of skin is unnecessary, it may toughen the skin, and it stings if the spirit is not allowed to dry.

Subcutaneous insulin is absorbed at different rates from different sites of the body. Soluble insulin has been found to be absorbed more effectively from the abdomen than from the thigh (Bartle et al., 1993). It is important therefore to use areas within one site at a certain time of the day in order to reliably predict the effectiveness of an insulin dose. For example, if insulin is usually injected into the abdomen in the morning, the thigh should not be used at this time. However, areas should be rotated within the site, and patients encouraged to use both left and right sides of the body.

The suitability of arms is currently being reviewed, and they are not usually recommended now as a first choice. If the arms are selected for injection a short needle should be used.

Patients should be encouraged to rotate their injection sites to prevent lipohypertrophy (lumps) which may make insulin absorption and therefore blood glucose levels erratic.

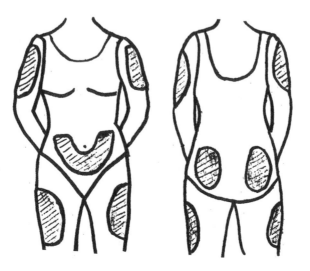

Figure 4.1: Injection sites front (left) and back (right)

At this stage it is usually a good idea to break for a cup of tea and some food. It is at least 30 minutes since insulin has been injected and a lot of information has been given.

Length of needle

Needles are available in lengths of 5 mm, 6 mm, 8 mm and 12.7 mm. It is suggested that children and adolescents should use 5 mm or 6 mm needles without a skin fold (although a skin fold can be used if preferred), and the same is recommended for thin adults. Normal weight adults should use 8 mm needles with a lifted skin fold; overweight adults should use a 12.7 mm needle with a lifted skin fold, or an 8 mm needle without the lifted skin fold (based on Strauss et al., 1999).

Storage of insulin

The insulin in use is stable at room temperature, away from radiators and direct sunlight, for one month. Insulin vials not in use should be stored in the fridge, not the freezer.

Free prescriptions

Those on insulin are exempt from prescription charges. Many patients are initially concerned about how they will afford treatment.

Identification (ID)

An ID card should be given; at a later stage ID bracelets and necklaces should be discussed (see pages 140–1).

Timing of injections

Insulin should be taken 20–30 minutes before food (5–15 minutes if analogue insulin). If food is delayed longer than this hypoglycaemia may occur.

Food

On day 1 only very little dietary advice is necessary. It is important to determine what the patient usually eats and base advice on this. Three regular meals containing carbohydrate should be eaten, and a snack before bed. Obvious sugar in drinks and sweets should be stopped. Ideally the patient should meet the dietitian and have an appointment within the first week of diagnosis.

Hypoglycaemia

Very small amounts of insulin are usually given initially; hypoglycaemia is therefore very unlikely providing the patient eats regularly. It is no longer considered good practice to induce hypoglycaemia. It is usually sufficient on day 1 to explain that a 'hypo' is a potential side-effect of insulin therapy. The aim of insulin therapy is to reduce the high levels of glucose or sugar in the blood; if the dose of insulin is too high for the amount of food eaten, or if exercise is taken, the level of glucose can fall to below normal. Symptoms to look out for are dizziness, light-headedness, tingling around the mouth, hunger or headache (see pp. 119–20). Dextrose tablets should be given to the patient, who should be advised to take three tablets in the event of a hypo followed by a biscuit, bread or cereal. Hypoglycaemia and its symptoms should be discussed more fully each day. It is important to reassure the patient that this is very unlikely to occur during the first few days. Additional information about hypoglycaemia should be given over the next few weeks.

Depending on how well the patient is feeling, how well he or she appears to be digesting the information, and the time of day, testing may be taught. However, the most important issues are that the patient is confident and able to administer insulin before the evening meal, is able to eat regularly and could treat hypoglycaemia. A simple written list of what to do until the next morning should be given to the patient, with an emergency phone number to be used if he or she has problems.

Box 4.2: Priorities for Day 1

(1) Explain what diabetes is and why insulin is necessary
(2) Teach injection technique:
  • How to inject
  • How to draw up using a syringe or dial up dose using a pen
  • How much to inject
  • Where to inject
  • When to inject
(3) Advice on storage of insulin
(4) Discuss what to eat and when, and refer to dietitian
(5) Provide ID card
(6) Discuss recognition and treatment of hypos
(7) Provide simple written information about what to do and how to do it
(8) Give emergency phone number

If there is time and the patient is able to take in more information, blood testing may be taught

---

Testing

During the first day the patient will have experienced capillary blood glucose monitoring either at his or her general practice or in casualty and most certainly by the DSN. These tests are an excellent opportunity for education; the procedure and the reasons for doing it should be explained and the patient involved as much as possible. I commonly perform a capillary blood glucose before insulin is given, and a couple of hours later to assess its effect. An opportunity is given for patients to 'have a go' at the second test. I usually demonstrate the procedure on myself before the second test, explaining each stage, and then talk the patient through the technique. Technique can be evaluated and revised at each visit over the next few weeks.

Home blood glucose monitoring (HBGM)

The ability to test blood glucose levels at home has enabled newly diagnosed Type 1 diabetes to be managed on an outpatient basis. HBGM demonstrates the effectiveness of insulin adjustments and can detect hypoglycaemia. Diabetes UK have coined the phrase 'make four the floor' recommending that blood glucose levels should not fall below 4 mmol/L. The only definitive method of diagnosing hypoglycaemia is by testing the blood glucose level. Newly diagnosed patients in particular may have become accustomed to hyperglycaemia and should be warned that they may feel 'hypo' at normal blood glucose levels or even at levels slightly higher than normal. It is therefore good practice to advise patients to test their blood glucose if they feel 'different' or unwell. Patients should be reassured that blood glucose levels of 4 mmol/L or above do not require treatment with glucose or sugar. HBGM often gives patients confidence. Many of the newer meters take only seconds to give a result and the blood does not require wiping, making testing much more convenient.

On a longer-term basis HBGM allows patients to assess their own blood glucose control and allows independent decisions to be made about their treatment and lifestyle.

What levels should the patient aim for?

Ultimately good control – blood glucose levels between 4 and 8 mmol/L most of the time. However, patients need reassurance that this is not always possible to achieve. Blood glucose levels are bound to fluctuate, particularly initially.

Blood glucose levels can be measured either visually or by using meters. Meters are not available on prescription and their prices vary. The strips are, however, available on prescription. Devices which automatically prick the finger are available but again these are not on prescription although the lancets which fit into the devices are. Some centres provide free meters and finger-pricking devices to those with new Type 1 diabetes. Whatever method is chosen and whatever local policy exists, a number of factors are important to consider.

- Adjustments to insulin doses are made on the strength of the results. Inappropriate treatment could be given if the readings are inaccurate due to incorrect technique
- Pricking the finger is uncomfortable. The number of tests suggested should therefore reflect the number that are strictly needed.

Important tips for HBGM

(1) Patients' hands should be washed in warm water with soap; if this is not possible they should be wiped with a wet, soapy flannel. If this is not done, sugar

on the patient's fingers, e.g. after eating an apple, rather than glucose in their bloodstream will be measured. This has potentially dangerous consequences.

(2) The side and not the tip of the finger should be used to obtain blood; it is much less painful.

(3) The finger should be 'milked' or 'pumped', not squeezed. Squeezing acts in the same way as a tourniquet and prevents blood flow.

(4) It is vital that enough blood is obtained to cover the strip completely. Meters 'under-read' and therefore give inaccurate results if less blood is obtained.

(5) The manufacturer's instructions should be followed to the letter. Meters should be re-calibrated every time a new pot/box of strips is used. Failure to follow the instructions leads to inaccurate results.

(6) Results should be recorded in a diary provided by the hospital, or some patients may choose to 'download' results on to a PC. Some meters now have this facility and a number of formats for presentation of the results are available.

On the first evening one blood glucose measurement is the most that is necessary. On the second day and during the first week it may be useful for the patient to perform four tests a day, gradually reducing these to two a day and then one a day at varied times. Willey et al. (1993) argued that once-daily HBGM at a variable time of the day gave adequate information for clinical intervention and had the advantage of reducing the heavy demand on people with diabetes.

Testing urine for ketones

This is easy to perform. Using Ketostix involves dipping a stick into the urine, removing it and waiting 15 seconds before matching the stick against a colour chart which indicates whether the urine is negative to ketones or contains trace, small, moderate or large amounts. The Optimum Meter (Medisense UK) is able to provide blood ketone and blood glucose levels. It can indicate whether the ketone levels are negative, low, mid or high and testing can be performed in the same way as blood glucose monitoring. At diagnosis those with Type 1 diabetes usually have moderate/mid or large/high amounts of ketones. These usually disappear during the first few days of insulin treatment, often before any significant decrease is seen in blood glucose levels. It can therefore be encouraging for patients to record this, and also prepares them for ketone testing during intercurrent illness (see p. 136).

Day 2

This usually starts by seeing how the patient got on with last evening's injection and a discussion of any problems or questions he or she may have. If blood or urine tests were performed, results should be discussed and the technique evaluated and revised as necessary. If blood and urine testing were not taught on day 1 they should be taught on day 2.

Driving

The DVLA must be informed if diabetes is treated with insulin. The doctor caring for the diabetes will be contacted to certify fitness to drive, and a licence will be issued for three years if no problems are identified. Licences may be issued for one-, two- or three-year periods. If patients experience loss of hypoglycaemic awareness, driving must stop until it is confirmed that symptoms have returned. If frequent episodes of hypoglycaemia are experienced, driving should cease until control is re-established; this will need confirmation by a doctor experienced in diabetes. Those with Type 1 diabetes are unable to hold heavy goods vehicle (HGV) or public service vehicle (PSV) licences. From 1 January 1998 the driving entitlements of people treated with insulin changed. The second EC Driving Licence Directive (91/439) prevented all persons on insulin from driving vehicles over 3.5 tonnes. Diabetes UK challenged this 'blanket ban' which had major adverse effects on employment for a substantial number of people on insulin. In April 2001, the government introduced a new legislation allowing people with insulin-treated diabetes to apply for the C1 licence needed to drive vans and small lorries between 3.5 and 7.5 tonnes – subject to individual assessment by a consultant. The ban on people with insulin-treated diabetes driving HGVs, minibuses and PSVs remains in force.

The insurance company should also be informed. Loading the premium should not occur because of diabetes; if it does, this should be challenged with the help of Diabetes UK's Diabetes Care and Information Service or a quote can be sought from Diabetes UK's insurance services.

Diabetes UK Motor Insurance
Tel: 0800 731 7432
Monday to Friday 8 am to 8 pm
Saturday 9 am to 3 pm

Reuse of syringes

It has previously been recommended that disposable syringes and pen needles can be reused safely up to five times. However, Becton Dickinson (needle manufacturers), who have always recommended single use of insulin needles, have now produced more compelling evidence for single use. Reuse leads to needle tip damage and loss of lubricant, which will increase pain and discomfort, and excessive use may lead to the microscopic end of the needle tip being broken off. This fact, together with pen needles now being available on prescription, has led many DSNs to recommend single use of pen needles.

Disposal of sharps

Local authorities vary widely with regard to the provision and collection of sharps boxes. Some provide and collect boxes – others do not! The health authority in which I work does not. Patients are therefore advised to use a Becton Dickinson (BD) Safeclip device which clips the tops off needles. The device stores about 1000 needles. Once the needle has been clipped, the cap should be replaced on the syringe and the syringe placed in an empty bleach or fabric conditioner bottle. When these are three-quarters full they can be disposed of in the domestic rubbish.

During the first few weeks

How to obtain supplies

Initial supplies of insulin, testing strips, injection devices, etc. are supplied by the DSN. Long-term supplies are obtained from the GP on prescription. A letter is written to the GP describing the insulin used and items needed and a list is also given to the patient.

Diet

For a full description see Chapter 2. An individual dietary assessment and prescription by a dietitian are necessary. The dietitian will explain the importance of eating regular amounts of food and how to swap carbohydrates. She or he will educate and advise about ideal body weight, alcohol, foods to eat during exercise or illness and will discuss any individual problems, such as eating disorders.

Mixing insulin / use of pens

Some centres may choose to manage those with Type 1 diabetes with twice-daily isophane or pre-mixed insulin for a few weeks or months. Long term, most with Type 1 diabetes need more flexibility than these regimes can offer (see p. 43). Those with Type 1 diabetes most commonly need either free-mixed insulin, e.g. Humulin S and Humulin I, Actrapid and Insulatard or a basal bolus regime, e.g. Humalog, Actrapid or Humulin S pre-meals and isophane insulin before bed using a pen.

Appendix 2 illustrates how to mix insulin if a twice-daily free-mixed regime is chosen. The procedure should be demonstrated and broken down into stages. The doses used should be as simple as possible, i.e. units of 5. A simple acronym may help some remember the order in which to draw up the air: ACAS:

Air
in
Cloudy
Air
in
Soluble (Clear)

followed by drawing up:

Clear
and then
Cloudy
Insulin

This can be written down for patients in addition to providing an illustrated booklet which describes each of the stages involved.

If a pen is chosen, patients should be given the opportunity to handle it, change the needle and change the cartridge (if necessary). A spare pen should always be given. Many pens are now available on prescription and spare pens can be obtained from GPs, if not available on prescription (e.g. Humapen Ergo). The DSN should provide a spare one. It is important that the patient is advised to perform an 'air shot' before each use to ensure that the pen is functioning correctly.

The benefit of introducing one of these regimes within the first couple of weeks is that patients can become involved in insulin adjustment. Each change in dose provides an excellent opportunity for education and the patient can be involved in decisions. By doing this, we aim to promote the idea that insulin adjustment can be undertaken by patients, not just professionals, and hope to encourage patients to take on this responsibility.

The honeymoon period

It may be necessary to reduce insulin doses fairly quickly after diagnosis to prevent hypoglycaemia during the 'honeymoon period'. During this time beta cells recover and begin to produce insulin again. This may last up to six months or a year. Patients should be warned about this as otherwise they are likely to feel that the diagnosis of Type 1 diabetes was a mistake and that they have been cured. During this period diabetes is often very easy to control and it provides a good opportunity for the patient to get used to diabetes. Insulin injections are not usually stopped during this time, although tiny doses are often all that is necessary. It is felt that continued insulin injections prolong beta cell function, and may also be easier psychologically. The honeymoon period usually ends abruptly during a bad cold or other stress to the beta cells.

The management of intercurrent illness

For a full description, see Chapter 5. Patients with Type 1 diabetes should be taught never to stop their insulin, even if they do not feel like eating. Usual meals should be replaced by liquid carbohydrate such as Lucozade if the patient is unable to eat normally. Blood glucose should be measured four times a day and the urine/blood tested for ketones at least twice a day. Insulin doses should be increased as necessary. If the patient is vomiting, and moderate/mid or large/high amounts of ketones are present or they feel increasingly symptomatic they should be advised to attend the Accident and Emergency Department.

Hypoglycaemia

Hypoglycaemia should be more fully discussed than it was on the first day. Fox and Pickering (1995) state that at a national youth conference 22 per cent of participants admitted to being 'terrified of hypoglycaemia'. Fox and Pickering also claim that those who hold a driving licence may be reluctant to describe or discuss hypos with the doctor responsible for certifying their capacity to drive.

Hypoglycaemia is defined as a plasma glucose concentration of below 3.3 mmol/L, although Diabetes UK now recommend that blood glucose levels should not fall below 4 mmol/L. However, clinically hypoglycaemia is more difficult to recognize (Appleton and Jerreat, 1995). As blood glucose falls below the normal range, a neuroendocrine response is generated. Counter-regulatory hormones – adrenaline, noradrenaline, glucagon and growth hormone – are released which cause a rapid release of glucose from the liver. This influences the clinical picture.

Symptoms

The symptoms of hypoglycaemia, although clearly listed in professional textbooks and patient education literature, may be different in practice and vary between individuals.

Table 4.1: Possible signs and symptoms of hypoglycaemia

Sweating	Trembling	Palpitations
Hunger	Tingling in hands/lips/tongue	Pallor
Blurred vision	Dizziness	Nausea
Headache	Weakness/tiredness	Slurred speech
Difficulty in concentrating	Bad temper/aggressiveness	Change in behaviour
Confusion	Fits	Paralysis/hemiplegia
	Loss of consciousness	

Nocturnal hypoglycaemia may be asymptomatic and recognizable only by night sweats and a headache on waking, accompanied by a high blood glucose level. If nocturnal hypoglycaemia is suspected, patients should be advised to perform a blood test at 2–3 am. If confirmed, evening doses of insulin can be reduced.

Patients usually rely on the early warning signs such as sweating, trembling and palpitations. These 'flight and fright' symptoms may be significantly reduced with increasing duration of diabetes, as can the glucagon response to hypoglycaemia.

Those with tightly controlled diabetes were found to have three times as many episodes of hypoglycaemia as those without tight control (DCCT, 1993). Those with tight control do not experience hypoglycaemic warning signs until their blood glucose levels are low. There is therefore more susceptibility to cerebral dysfunction, which may in turn render them incapable of taking action. Lack of warning may also be related to the speed at which the blood glucose falls. Loss of symptoms due to tight control can be reversed by running blood glucose at higher levels and stopping all hypos.

It has been suggested that human insulin may cause hypoglycaemic unawareness. Little evidence has been found worldwide to substantiate this (BDA, 1991). However, if patients wish to change to animal sources of insulin this should be done without fuss.

Autonomic neuropathy may lead to hypoglycaemic unawareness as symptoms such as sweating, tremor and palpitations are mediated by the autonomic nervous system. Those with severe autonomic damage should therefore run higher blood glucose levels. Treatment with betablockers may also lead to a lack of symptoms.

Box 4.3: Causes of hypoglycaemia

- Too much insulin
- Inadequate amounts of carbohydrate
- Delayed/missed meals
- Unplanned or sustained exercise
- Incorrect timings of insulin
- Alcohol
- Honeymoon period
- Change of injection site

Hypoglycaemia caused by exercise or alcohol can occur several hours later. The effects of alcohol may also mask hypoglycaemic symptoms.

Prevention

- Regular meals and snacks (particularly if on twice-daily insulin). If a meal is delayed an additional snack should be taken.
- Insulin should be taken 20–30 minutes before meals, with the exception of analogues which should be taken 5–15 minutes before meals. A longer delay could lead to hypoglycaemia.
- Monitor blood glucose levels regularly to establish suitability of insulin dose.
- Eat before driving; do not drive if a meal is due. Check blood glucose level before long journeys and make regular stops for food. Carry carbohydrate in the car; if a hypo does occur turn off the engine, get out of the driving seat and remove the keys from the ignition.

- If exercise is planned, decrease insulin or increase carbohydrate; if exercise is unplanned, increase carbohydrate (see p. 146).
- Limit alcohol intake (see p. 143). Ensure a bedtime snack containing carbohydrate is taken.
- Discourage 'stat' doses of insulin in response to a single high blood glucose (chasing tail) see p. 45).
- If injection sites are changed from lipohypertrophic sites, insulin doses should be decreased as absorption from the sites will improve.
- Carry glucose tablets or some form of rapidly acting carbohydrate.
- Carry identification and educate workmates/friends.
- Those with hypoglycaemic unawareness may benefit from systems such as the Glucowatch (see p. 127), which has an alarm that sounds if blood glucose falls and CSII pump therapy (see p. 49) which has been shown to reduce hypoglycaemia. However both of these are expensive and the cost may need to be met at least in part by the individual.

Treatment

Ideally a blood glucose reading should be performed; treatment is required if the blood glucose is less than 4 mmol/L. Treatment will usually depend on the severity of the symptoms.

If 'mild' symptoms such as sweating, tingling of the lips, hunger or slight trembling are experienced, a form of quick-acting carbohydrate should be taken such as three dextrose tablets, two teaspoons of sugar or a glass of milk.

If symptoms are more severe or if the person is confused or aggressive, liquid forms of carbohydrate such as ordinary Coca Cola, fruit juice or Lucozade are preferable as these act more quickly.

If symptoms do not improve after 5–10 minutes treatment should be repeated. After treatment with quick-acting carbohydrate when symptoms have resolved, a high-fibre snack or a meal containing carbohydrate should be taken to prevent recurrence.

Severe hypoglycaemia is characterized by unconsciousness and possibly fitting. Food and drink must not be given. Hypostop or Glucagon (available on prescription) can be used by relatives or friends. Those with Type 1 diabetes and their family should be provided with these and taught how to use them.

- Hypostop is a dextrose gel administered orally and is rapidly absorbed through the buccal mucosa.
- Glucagon comes in a kit. It can be administered by subcutaneous injection and causes release of glucose from the liver.

If Hypostop and glucagon are ineffective, intravenous glucose is necessary. If this occurs, an ambulance should be called.

Smoking

Stopping smoking is one of the most positive things that can be done to reduce the risk of diabetic complications. Smoking doubles the risk of vascular disease (BDA, 1996/97). In terms of coronary heart disease Fox and Pickering (1995) argue that stopping smoking is better than any other intervention and would prolong by three years the life of the average 45-year-old man with diabetes. Patients often find it difficult to make the connection between foot problems and smoking and therefore education is required to help them do this. The BDA (1996/97) claim that giving up smoking actually reduced the risk of limb amputation by 26 times in women with diabetes.

'Stop smoking groups' may be available at GP surgeries or health education units. Quitline, a national phone helpline which provides expert advice, information packs and details of local groups, may be helpful.

• Quitline, Tel: 0800 002200; Answerphone outside office hours

Footcare

This will be covered in detail in the section, 'Education of those with Type 2 diabetes'.

Recreational drugs

There is little written information about the effects of these drugs.

Smoking 'dope' (cannabis and marijuana) may increase blood glucose levels and increase hunger. Ecstasy too, tends to increase blood glucose levels and can lead to ketoacidosis. Dehydration may be a contributory factor. Increased exercise at raves should decrease blood glucose. Amphetamines (speed) and cocaine can lead to a high energy expenditure, so provoking hypoglycaemia and decreasing appetite. Patients should be encouraged not to stop insulin in an attempt to prevent hypos due to the risk of DKA. Advice if taking ecstasy would therefore usually be to increase carbohydrate and fluid intake but not to reduce insulin doses.

Complications

It is always a difficult decision when and how to address the subject of long-term complications; however, I believe that the subject should not be avoided. Often patients have heard horror stories about the effects of diabetes and addressing these fears and giving up-to-date and correct information does much to build trust and respect between the patient and professional.

The results of the DCCT (see pp. 60–3) can be used to encourage patients. It demonstrated that tight blood glucose control (HbA1$_c$ levels of around 7 per cent) decreased the development and progression of retinopathy, neuropathy and nephropathy by an average of about 60 per cent. It demonstrated that any improvement in control has a positive impact on complications. It is, however, important to acknowledge the difficulties involved in controlling diabetes and the huge amount of support available to participants in the study. As previously discussed, the risk of hypoglycaemia increases, as does the risk of weight gain.

Patients should be reassured that regular screening can detect problems at an early stage. Many of these, such as background retinopathy and microalbuminuria can be treated effectively. Complications should never be used as a threat, i.e. if you don't do this you will go blind. It is not helpful and may not be true. It is also vitally important to make it clear that it is not the patient's fault if complications occur. Good control reduces the risk by 60 per cent, not 100 per cent; there are no promises, just reduced risks.

Effects of diabetes on employment

Some jobs have blanket bans preventing employment of those with Type 1 diabetes, although for those already employed in these occupations it is usual to be offered an alternative job within the organization. The BDA (1996/97) argues that blanket bans are often long-standing practices and may be the result of outdated ideas about diabetes. Examples of jobs with blanket bans are the armed forces, airline pilot, cabin crew with most airlines, fire and police service, train driver and any job which requires an HGV or PSV licence. The BDA (1996/97) cites the blanket ban for working offshore as an example of an illogical ban. It includes working for most cruise liners and means that even a caterer with Type 1 diabetes would not pass the offshore certificate.

Patients may need a letter of support from the diabetes team to give to their employers, particularly if they feel that they have been refused a job which does not carry a blanket ban. Diabetes UK encourages people to appeal if they feel that they have been refused employment in an area which does not carry a blanket restriction solely on the grounds of diabetes. They also advise seeking help from the local Citizens' Advice Bureau and union representatives if patients are already employed and are moved to another job or discharged on medical grounds.

Patients should be advised to be honest about their condition and tell both their employers and work colleagues about their diabetes. Short breaks for snacks and regular meals are usually necessary and colleagues will need to know what to do in case of hypos. But it is important that diabetes is not used as an excuse to avoid work.

A booklet entitled Employment and Diabetes (code 9108) is available from Diabetes UK: cost £1.30.

How to cope with exercise/eating out

Exercise should be encouraged and people helped with food/insulin adjustment as necessary (see Chapter 5 for more information).

Eating out may involve changing insulin doses and timing. The patient should be reassured that there is always a way to handle this. Patients should be helped and encouraged to alter insulin doses and times, earlier rather than later.

Diabetes UK (formerly the British Diabetic Association)

Diabetes UK is a self-help charity which has people with diabetes and their families and friends and health care professionals as members. A confidential telephone careline is provided between the hours of 9 am and 5 pm Monday to Friday, and is open to both members and non-members. Diabetes UK organizes holidays for children and teenagers and a youth diabetic project for 18- to 35-year-olds with a quarterly newsletter. It provides many leaflets (some free) and *Balance*, a bi-monthly magazine, is provided free to members. Diabetes UK organizes conferences for both professionals and patients and organizes research into the causes and treatment of diabetes. It provides a powerful voice within the health care system and at government level. In the 1980s the BDA secured free 'disposable' syringes and blood testing strips for those with diabetes. Diabetes UK has more recently campaigned to secure pen needles on prescription and an assurance by the pharmaceutical industry that animal insulins will continue to be produced.

The cost of membership tends to vary from year to year and concessions are made for pensioners, students, children and those receiving DSS grants.

Travel advice

This is covered in detail in Chapter 5.

Section Three: The Education of those with Type 2 Diabetes

Barriers to education

Walker (1993) claims that because many people with Type 2 diabetes fall into the 65 plus age-group they may have specific barriers to learning. She cites these as (1) visual and or auditory impairment; (2) well-established habits, especially eating patterns; (3) impressions of diabetes from long ago; (4) other medical conditions; (5) they may not have been in a learning situation for many years. In addition to these factors, Type 2 diabetes is more common in those from ethnic minority groups for whom English may not be their first language and who differ in cultural beliefs (see Chapter 6, pp. 161–7).

Education programmes need to be planned taking these factors into account.

Serious nature of Type 2 diabetes

It is vital that patients are aware that Type 2 diabetes is not 'mild' diabetes, as it has often been called in the past. Mild diabetes gives the impression that it does not warrant much care and attention, either by patients in terms of lifestyle modification or by professionals. Type 2 diabetes can give rise to serious complications (see Chapter 3), particularly if preventive measures and screening have not been adopted.

Type 2 diabetes does not disappear

Many people with Type 2 diabetes feel that their diabetes will go away. Unfortunately I have encountered patients who, because of negative home urine tests and relief of symptoms, stopped attending screening clinics, stopped testing and stopped dieting only to be referred back 15 years later with established complications of diabetes.

Diet

Dietary modification is important for those with Type 2 diabetes, particularly those who are overweight. The reduction of saturated fats is considered most important to reduce the incidence of cardiovascular disease. Dietitians should be involved in education and may use 'The Balance of Good Health' model recommended by the Health Education Authority (1995) to teach healthy eating. The model uses a plate divided into five food groups: (1) fruit and vegetables; (2) bread, cereals and potatoes; (3) milk and dairy foods; (4) fatty and sugary foods; and (5) meat, fish and alternatives. It suggests the amounts from each group which should be taken.

Oral hypoglycaemic agents

Please see Chapter 2 for a full discussion. Type 2 diabetes is a progressive disease; the majority of patients will need tablets and 30 per cent may need insulin therapy. Patients should be warned about this at diagnosis. Tablet and insulin therapy should not be used as threats; patients are not failures if they need tablets or insulin. It is important to explain that the treatment and not the patient has failed.

Patients should be informed of the actions and side-effects of all oral hypoglycaemics. They should be involved in the decision about which are most suitable for them. Full information should also be given on how and when the tablets should be taken and the precautions necessary, e.g. to take increased carbohydrate if increased exercise is taken when treated with sulphonylureas.

Testing

Monitoring of diabetes helps the professional to advise on therapy. Most importantly though, it can help patients to regain control over their lives and take responsibility for their diabetes management. The effects of different foods and activities can be assessed, and improving blood or urine test results can be a source of great encouragement to patients to continue with the diet.

For those with Type 2 diabetes a choice between either blood or urine testing needs to be made. Patients should be advised of the advantages and disadvantages of each method and helped to make an informed decision on which is best for them and their circumstances. In practice most people choose to blood test in the unit where I work, possibly because a meal is provided free of charge.

Patients need to understand the benefits for them of monitoring. If they do not they are unlikely to perform the tests. The professional needs to ensure that there are benefits for the patient. For example, if a person is frail and very elderly without other serious medical conditions, is control of symptoms alone not enough?

Is the patient capable of doing the test? Considerations such as sight, dexterity, the ability to record and understand the results and whether the patient or the professional will act on the results should be weighed up. The cost to the NHS should also be considered. Using blood glucose strips is considerably more expensive than testing urine; though this should not be a barrier to their prescription to those who will use them effectively, they should not be wasted.

Whichever method patients choose, this should be demonstrated by the professional, the technique broken down into stages and opportunities given for patients to practise.

Home urine testing (HUT)

Advantages

(1) Simple to perform, which makes the technique likely to be accurately performed.
(2) Painless, which may encourage patients to perform regular tests.

Disadvantages

(1) It is unable to detect hypoglycaemia.
(2) It gives only a crude indication of blood glucose control as it reflects what has been happening to the glucose in the bladder since the bladder was last emptied.
(3) It is reliant on renal threshold. The renal threshold is the level at which glucose overflows from the blood into the urine. The usual level for adults is 10 mmol/L. This can, however, vary; the renal threshold may be higher or lower.

High renal threshold

This means that blood glucose levels are substantially higher than 10 mmol/L before glucose overflows into the urine. Patients will therefore have negative HUT despite high blood glucose and HbA1$_c$ levels. Before concluding that the patient has a high renal threshold, the nurse should check that the patient is performing the test correctly and that he or she is performing post-prandial (after food) tests in additional to fasting tests. A common reason for negative results is tests performed only when fasting or on 'good' days.

Low renal threshold

A low renal threshold would be suspected if HUT measurements were always positive despite excellent control measured by blood glucose and HbA1$_c$ readings.

If the patient has a high or low renal threshold, HUT is inaccurate and HBGM is necessary.

Home blood glucose monitoring (HBGM)

Advantages

(1) Direct rather than indirect measurement of blood glucose at a precise time.
(2) Able to detect hypoglycaemia.

Disadvantages

(1) It is painful. This may make it unacceptable to some, who may perform very few tests, which may therefore provide little information.
(2) It is more complicated to perform.
(3) Incorrect technique can lead to vastly inaccurate results.

Urine

It is rarely necessary for those with Type 2 diabetes to test more than once a day, except during intercurrent illness. If diabetes is well controlled, two or three times a week is usually all that is necessary. If the urine is tested it is usually recommended that some tests are performed two hours after the largest meal. When newly diagnosed, daily tests may be helpful to demonstrate to patients that treatment is effective.

HBGM should be performed at varied times of the day. One blood glucose test a day performed at varied times each day is more valuable than two tests a day performed at the same times every day.

Meters

A variety of blood glucose meters and lancet devices are available which can be purchased either directly from manufacturers or from retail pharmacies. DSNs are also often given free samples to distribute to patients who would benefit from meters.

Two new methods of blood glucose monitoring have recently been launched. One is the soft-sense 'all-in-one-step' blood glucose testing meter/lancet device. This allows testing to be carried out on sites other than fingers (e.g. the forearm or upper arm) which are less sensitive than fingers. The other is the Glucowatch which is worn like a watch and takes non invasive glucose readings through the skin every 20 minutes for 12 hours at a time. It has a built-in alarm which can indicate high, low and rapidly changing blood glucose levels. However, capillary blood glucose readings are necessary to calibrate the device, perspiration may cause the watch to stop monitoring, and you are unable to shower, bath or swim whilst wearing it! The low level electric current can cause skin irritation and blistering. Both these devices are also expensive – the soft-sense is currently £225.00 and the Glucowatch £350.00. Autosensors for the Glucowatch are not available on prescription and cost £50 for 16; lancets and strips for the soft-sense device are both available on prescription.

Driving

Those managed on diet alone need not notify the DVLA unless they develop eye problems which affect visual acuity or visual fields.

For Group II entitlement they must notify the DVLA and their medical condition will be reviewed. They will be licensed unless visual complications develop.

Those managed by tablets must notify the DVLA. If medical enquiries are satisfactory the licence can be kept until aged 70 years unless eye problems develop. For Group II entitlement the DVLA must be notified; drivers will be licensed if a medical examination is satisfactory.

Smoking (see p. 122)

Footcare

A brief and simple explanation of why diabetes can affect the feet is necessary. For example, diabetes can affect the feet for two main reasons: (1) diabetes can affect the blood vessels, leading to poor circulation to the feet and legs. Blood supply is needed to keep the tissues healthy and supplied with oxygen. Smoking can make blood circulation worse; (2) diabetes can cause damage to the nerves, which may cause numbness or tingling. Pain is our biggest protection against injury, therefore if areas on the feet cannot be felt injuries can occur without people being aware of them and infection can quickly develop.

It is important to discuss horror stories and dispel myths. Most foot problems are preventable with good foot care.

It is a good idea for patients to have their feet assessed and be aware of any ischaemia or neuropathy. This can be done either in the hospital diabetic clinic or at the general practice, and ideally also by a state-registered chiropodist who will provide footcare advice specific to the patient.

General footcare advice

Feet should be washed at least once a day with soap and warm water and carefully dried afterwards, particularly between the toes. Pure cotton or woollen socks should be worn. Feet should be examined daily; a mirror should be used if the soles of the feet cannot be seen easily. Any change in colour, for example redness, could indicate infection even in the absence of pain. Any swelling, weeping or strange smells could indicate infection. Infection is always serious with diabetes and immediate medical attention and antibiotics are essential.

Hard skin should be prevented and treated using pumice stones and files and hand cream or E45 cream applied. Cracks in hard skin provide an entry site for infection and require chiropody treatment. Corns should not be treated with corn plasters, which contain acid and can burn, leading to ulcers and infection, nor should 'do it yourself' surgery be performed. Toenails should be cut either to the shape of the toe or straight across and after washing the feet when they are softer. Shoes should fit properly and new shoes should be worn in gradually, examining feet frequently for blisters. Chiropodists can advise on suitable shoes and local shops which measure and fit shoes properly.

Intercurrent illness

Please see Chapter 5.

Complications

Unlike those with Type 1 diabetes, some with newly diagnosed Type 2 diabetes already have established complications of diabetes. Support for, and treatment of, complications are therefore needed. Many have Type 2 diabetes long before it is detected. The major cause of death for those with Type 2 diabetes is macrovascular complications, namely heart disease. Hypertension in those with this type of diabetes is associated with a twofold risk of heart attack and a threefold risk of stroke and amputation compared with normotensive people with Type 2 diabetes (Fox and Pickering, 1995). Blood pressure must therefore be controlled. Patients should be encouraged to stop smoking, reduce salt intake and limit alcohol intake. The intake of saturated fat should be reduced and attempts made to achieve a healthy weight for height and take some form of exercise. Foot, eye and renal complications should also be discussed (see Chapter 3).

What diabetes care to expect

Diabetes UK publishes a free leaflet describing the care that patients with both Type 2 and Type 1 diabetes should expect at diagnosis and once diabetes is controlled. It describes the types of care available, i.e. GP clinics, mini clinics, hospital clinics or by community services. The benefits and drawbacks of each type of clinic will be addressed in Chapter 8. Most importantly the leaflet contains what patients should expect from an annual review. All patients should have access to this leaflet to help them to ensure that they are receiving this care. The reason that each investigation is necessary should be explained; please see suggested explanations in parentheses.

At the annual review

- Weight should be recorded (this is a useful way of monitoring diabetes control and the success of treatment). If weight should be decreasing and it is, treatment is working. If too much weight has been lost, diabetes may be poorly controlled. Weight gain may indicate overtreatment with medication or failure to understand and/or follow the diet.

- Urine should be tested for protein (indication of infection or kidney disease).
- Blood should be tested to measure long-term control, i.e. HbA1$_c$ or fructosamine (provides an average blood glucose level), and urea and electrolytes for renal function and lipids should also be checked.
- An opportunity should be given for discussion, which should include blood or urine test results.
- The blood pressure should be checked (high blood pressure increases the risk of heart disease, strokes and kidney and eye disease). If blood pressure is found to be more than 140/80, treatment should be given.
- Vision should be checked and the back of the eye examined; drops are inserted to make viewing easier. A photograph may also be taken.
- Legs and feet (without shoes and socks) should be examined to check blood and nerve supply. If problems are identified, referral to a chiropodist should be made.
- Opportunity should be given to discuss how diabetes is affecting work and home life and feelings.

The NSF for diabetes (DoH, 2003) recommends that a personal diabetes record that contains the clinical record of treatment and management (including test results) should be held by the person with diabetes. It should include an agreed care plan incorporating education, patient goals and an explanation of how diabetes care will be met, and by whom. Copies of all correspondence about the patient should be given to them.

Travel/holiday advice

Please see Chapter 5.

Diabetes Education: A Summary

- Information should be given according to the specific needs of the patient and in the order that he or she wants it.
- It should be simple to understand with no jargon.
- Small amounts of information should be given at a time, building on current knowledge.
- Written information should reinforce oral information whenever possible. This should be clear and simple to understand, but not patronizing.
- Leaflets/videos/software should be in the patient's preferred language.
- Information should be consistent and accurate.
- Practical skills should be demonstrated and time allocated in which patients can practise.
- Patient understanding should be regularly evaluated before more information is given.

Box 4.4: NSF Standards (DoH, 2001b)

Standard 3: Empowering people with diabetes

(3) All children, young people and adults with diabetes will receive a service which encourages partnership in decision-making, supports them in managing their diabetes and helps them to adopt and maintain a healthy lifestyle. This will be reflected in an agreed and shared care plan in an appropriate format and language. Where appropriate, parents and carers should be fully engaged in this process.

Standards 5 and 6: Clinical care of children and young people with diabetes

(5) All children and young people with diabetes will receive consistently high-quality care and they, with their families, and others involved in their day-to-day care, will be supported to optimize the control of their blood glucose and their physical, psychological, intellectual, educational and social development.

(6) All young people with diabetes will experience a smooth transition of care from paediatric diabetes services to adult diabetes services, whether hospital or community based, either directly or via a young people's clinic. The transition will be organized in partnership with each individual and at an age appropriate to and agreed with them.

Standard 7: Management of diabetic emergencies

(7) The NHS will develop, implement and monitor agreed protocols for rapid and effective treatment of diabetic emergencies by appropriately trained health care professionals. Protocols will include the management of acute complications and procedures to minimize the risk of recurrence.

Standard 8: Care of people with diabetes during admission to hospital

(8) All children, young people and adults with diabetes admitted to hospital, for whatever reason, will receive effective care of their diabetes. Whenever possible, they will continue to be involved in decisions concerning the management of their diabetes.

Standards 10, 11 and 12: Detection and management of long-term complications

(10) All young people and adults with diabetes will receive regular surveillance for the long-term complications of diabetes.

(11) The NHS will develop, implement and monitor agreed protocols and systems of care to ensure that all people who develop long-term complications of diabetes receive timely, appropriate and effective investigation and treatment to reduce their risk of disability and premature death.

(12) All people with diabetes requiring multi-agency support will receive integrated health and social care.

National Service Framework

The NSF standards relevant to this chapter are shown in Box 4.4.

Questions (one for each learning outcome)

(1) How should a health professional approach the education of a person with diabetes? Is telling them what to do enough?
(2) Sharon Neville was diagnosed with Type 1 diabetes one week ago. She and her partner Peter are concerned about hypoglycaemia and require further information. How would you approach this and what information would you give?
(3) Mr Batty has Type 2 diabetes and takes metformin 500 mg bd. He is not performing any type of home testing. What advice would you offer?

Suggested answers may be found on pages 253–4.

References

Almond J, Cox D, Nugent M, Day JL Rayman GR and Graham A (2001) Experience of group sessions for converting to insulin. Journal of Diabetes Nursing 5(4): 102–5.
Annersten M, Frid A (2000) Insulin pens dribble from the tip of the needle after injection. Practical Diabetes International 17(4): 109–11.
Appleton M, Jerreat L (1995) Hypoglycaemia. Nursing Standard 10(5): 37–42.
Bartle JP, Neal L, Frankamp LM (1993) Effects of the anatomical region used for insulin injections on glycaemia in Type 1 diabetes subjects. Diabetes Care 16(12): 1592–7.
Blaxter M (1983) Health services as a defence against the consequences of poverty in industralised societies. Social Science and Medicine 17(16): 1139–48.
British Diabetic Association (1991) Loss of Hypoglycaemia Warning Symptoms in the use of Human Insulins. Report from the LOW Taskforce. London: BDA.
British Diabetic Association (1996/97) Balance For Beginners Starting Out With Insulin Dependent Diabetes. London: BDA.
Coles C (1989) Diabetes education: theories of practice. Practical Diabetes 6(5): 199–201.
Day JL (1996) All this education: is it worthwhile? Practical Diabetes International 13(4): 125–7.
DCCT Research Group (1993) Diabetes Control and Complications Trial (DCCT): results of a feasibility study. Diabetes Care 10: 1–19.
Delaney F (1991) Getting the message across. Nursing 4(43): 24–5.
Department of Health (2001a) The Expert Patient. A New Approach to Chronic Disease Management for the 21st Century. London: HMSO.
Department of Health (2001b) The National Service Framework in Disease Standards. London: HMSO.
Department of Health (2003) The National Service Framework in Diabetes Delivery Strategy. London: HMSO.
Fox C, Pickering A (1995) Diabetes in the Real World. London: Class Publishing.
Fox J, Benzeval M (1995) Perspectives on social variations in health. In Benzeval M, Judge K, Smaje C (Eds) Beyond class, race and ethnicity: deprivation and health in Britain. Health Services Research Special Issue 30(1).

Graham H (1993) When Life's a Drag: Women, Smoking and Disadvantage. Department of Health. London: HMSO.

Health Educational Authority (1995) Changing What You Eat: The Balance of Good Health – A Plan For You. London: Health Education Authority.

Heller S (2001) Interim results from Dose Adjustment for Normal Eating (DAFNE) Programme. Journal of Diabetes Nursing 5(3): 94.

Jervell J (1996) Education is as important as insulin, oral drugs and proper food for people with diabetes. Practical Diabetes International 13(5): 142.

Kaplan RM, Chadwick MW, Schimmel LE (1985) Social learning intervention to promote metabolic control in Type 1 diabetes mellitus: pilot experiment results. Diabetes Care 8: 152–5.

Lockington TJ, Powles S, Meadows KA, Wise PH (1988) Attitudes, knowledge and blood glucose control. Diabetic Medicine 6: 309–13.

Shillitoe RW (1992) The complete diabetes educator. Practical Diabetes 9(1): 30.

Strauss K, Hannet I, McGonigie J, Parkes JL, Ginsberg B, Jamal R, Frid A (1999) Ultra-Short (5 mm) insulin needles: trial results and clinical recommendations. Practical Diabetes International 16(7): 218–22.

Townsend P, Whitehead M, Davidson N (Eds) (1992) Inequalities in Health: The Black Report and The Health Divide. New edn. Harmondsworth: Penguin.

Walker R (1993) The gentle art of giving information to people with Type 2 diabetes, part 1: An alternative to checklists. Practical Diabetes 10(3): 114–15.

Willey KA, Twigg SM, Constantino MI, Yue DK, Turtle JR (1993) Home blood glucose monitoring: how often? Practical Diabetes 10(1): 22–5.

World Health Organisation (1984) Health Promotion: A Discussion Document on the Concepts and Principles. Copenhagen: WHO Regional Office for Europe.

Chapter 5
Commonly occurring situations which make diabetes more difficult to control

This chapter discusses commonly occurring situations which can make diabetes more difficult to control and may require the adjustment of insulin or tablet therapy. The effects of intercurrent illness, travel and exercise will be addressed.

Learning Outcomes

After reading this chapter you should be able to:

(1) Educate those with Type 1 diabetes and Type 2 diabetes about how to cope with intercurrent illness, including the recognition of danger signs.
(2) Advise on safe travel and identify when to involve a diabetes specialist nurse (DSN) and/or doctor.
(3) Suggest how those with Type 1 and Type 2 diabetes can exercise without experiencing either hypo- or hyperglycaemia.

Intercurrent Illness

Illness can have dramatic effects on diabetes control. Diabetes is often poorly managed during acute intercurrent illness (Marsden and Grant, 1991), and many people treated with insulin are unaware that insulin should be continued when they are ill.

During infection, levels of counter-regulatory hormones, e.g. adrenaline, noradrenaline, glucagon, cortisol and growth hormone, rise in those both with and without diabetes. These hormones act directly on the liver, stimulating glycogen and fat breakdown and causing blood glucose to rise. In those without diabetes more insulin is produced to compensate and normal blood glucose levels are maintained. In those with diabetes, insulin levels cannot be increased, resulting in hyperglycaemia. Ketones may be produced in those with Type 1 diabetes.

134

People with Type 1 diabetes are totally dependent on injected insulin. If depleted of insulin, ketones are produced due to a breakdown of fat and muscle by the liver (gluconeogenesis). The accumulation of ketones is potentially dangerous and can lead to diabetic ketoacidosis (DKA).

Illnesses such as the common cold, urinary tract infections and flu can all affect diabetes. Steroid therapy also increases blood glucose levels. Amongst the most difficult of situations to manage is gastroenteritis, particularly if anorexia or vomiting occurs.

Before advice or education can be given about management of diabetes it is important to establish whether the person has Type 1 or Type 2 diabetes. Those who have Type 2 diabetes – whether treated by diet, diet and tablets or diet and insulin – can produce some insulin of their own, although an increase in treatment is usually required during illness.

Assessment

In order to determine the effects of illness, the severity of hyperglycaemic symptoms such as polydipsia, polyuria, nocturia and weight loss should be assessed. A random blood glucose and urinalysis should be performed. It is vital to determine whether the person with diabetes is able to eat normally and whether he or she is taking his or her diabetes tablets or insulin. It is also useful to assess the experience and the level of understanding the patient has of the management of diabetes during intercurrent illness.

General advice

- What to do when ill should be discussed before it happens, as part of routine education by the diabetes specialist nurse, the practice nurse, the GP or the hospital clinic. Ideally, written information should also be given.
- Prompt medical treatment, for example antibiotics, should be sought for infections (BDA, 1995a). Paracetamol or aspirin can be taken to relieve pyrexia if necessary.
- Cough mixtures and cold remedies should be sugar free.
- If possible the person should continue to eat normally. If unable to eat normally, meals should be replaced with soups, cereals or liquid carbohydrate (CHO). CHO must be taken even if blood glucose levels are elevated. It is a common mistake to withhold food if blood glucose is high, but this may make ketosis worse (Curry and Weedon, 1993).
- Plenty of sugar-free drinks should be taken; at least five pints a day.
- If vomiting occurs and the person is unable to tolerate liquid CHO, medical attention should be sought.
- Tablets and insulin should be continued, even if the person is not eating normally. It is important to ensure that medication is being taken at the correct times and in the correct dosages.
- The dosage of tablets or insulin may need to be increased. If tablets are being taken, care should be taken not to exceed the maximum dose. If the

maximum doses of tablets are being taken and the patient is symptomatic, particularly if the infection is severe or likely to be of long duration, insulin may be required for the duration of the infection.
- Blood (if on insulin) or urine should be tested for glucose at least four times a day. Those with Type 1 diabetes should also check for ketones.

Case-study 5.1 (Type 2 diabetes)

Mr Fred Jenkins is 60 years of age and has well-controlled Type 2 diabetes treated with gliclazide 80 mg bd and metformin 500 mg bd. He has 'the flu' and complains of polyuria, lethargy, polydipsia and nocturia four times a night. His urine tests contain 2 per cent glucose despite the fact that he is eating very little. His wife has suggested that he stop eating altogether and drink only water, that he should stop testing (as the results seemed to worry him), stop the medication (in case of hypoglycaemia) and go to bed.

The recommended treatment would include:

- Try to eat normally; if unable to do so substitute cereals, milk, soups or sugary drinks
- Test urine four times a day
- Increase gliclazide to a maximum of 160 mg bd over the next two to three days as necessary. As 'flu' subsides reduce gliclazide to the usual dose
- Ensure that any cough mixture or cold remedies are sugar free
- If the cough, or the control of diabetes, does not improve contact his GP.

Specific management of Type 1 diabetes during illness

The aim is to prevent diabetic ketoacidosis and to prevent symptoms of hyperglycaemia. Blood glucose should be tested and recorded at least four times a day, before breakfast, before lunch, before dinner and before bed. Urine/blood should be tested for ketones at least twice a day, four times a day if positive.

During illness the dose of insulin may need to be increased by between 25 per cent and 30 per cent. If the blood glucose is 13 mmol/L or less and there are no ketones, the patient should continue with the usual insulin doses. If blood glucose is higher and ketones are present, extra soluble insulin is required. Soluble insulin can safely be given every six hours. A DSN or doctor can give individual written information about how to increase insulin dosages before illness occurs (Figure 5.1). Ideally, advice should be based on the patient's usual insulin requirements. Prompt action may prevent the need for hospital admission.

Those with Type 1 diabetes are usually managed on a twice-daily free-mixing regime such as Humulin S and Humulin I or a four times a day basal bolus regime such as Actrapid tds and Insulatard nocte. This allows increased doses of soluble insulin to be given as necessary. If the patient usually takes pre-mixed or intermediate-acting insulin only, it may be necessary to add soluble insulin. Increases in dosage of intermediate-acting insulin should not be undertaken more frequently than at two- to three-day intervals (see p. 49).

Sick Day Rules

Never stop your insulin

Food
* If unable to eat solids, sip Lucozade, sugary coke or sugary lemonade, etc.
You must have <u>at least</u> one glass (200 ml/8 fl oz) for each meal.
e.g. 1 glass for breakfast to be sipped until lunchtime.

If unable to tolerate sugary drinks, or vomiting, come to Accident and Emergency.

Testing
* **Test blood sugar 4 times a day**
Before breakfast
Before lunch
Before evening meal
Before bed

* Test urine or blood for ketones at least twice a day (4 times if positive).

Action
* If blood sugar Is:
Less than 13, no extra insulin is needed.
13 or above, extra clear soluble insulin is necessary.
This can be given every 6 hours in addition to your normal dose.

If ketones are moderate/mid or large/high despite extra insulin, come to Accident and Emergency

Suggested amounts of extra .... (type of) insulin to be given;
If blood sugar is;		
	$13 \rightarrow 16.9$	give .... units
	$17 \rightarrow 19.9$	give .... units
	20 or above	give .... units
If ketones moderate or large		give .... units

Additional advice

Devised by Lynne Jerreat   Queen Elizabeth Hospital Healthcare Trust

Figure 5.1: Management of Type 1 diabetes during illness

As infection subsides, blood glucose will fall. If diabetes control was poor before the illness, increased doses of insulin may still be required and these should be added to the usual bd or basal bolus regime, rather than given as stat doses.

If the person with Type 1 diabetes is unable to eat normally, small amounts of liquid CHO should be sipped throughout the day. Liquid CHO contains no fibre and therefore causes blood glucose to rise and fall rapidly. At least one glass of Lucozade or a similar type of glucose drink should be taken to cover each meal.

Intercurrent illness in those with Type 1 diabetes requires skilful management. Although the principles are straightforward, both patients and health care professionals need to be aware of the danger signs that require urgent specialist attention.

Table 5.1: Danger signs

(1) Increasing blood glucose >17 mmol/L despite increased insulin doses
(2) Increasing symptoms of hyperglycaemia
(3) Vomiting. If unable to tolerate a glass of CHO containing fluid, intravenous fluids are necessary
(4) Moderate or large amounts of ketones in the urine

An ambulance and urgent admission to hospital are required if abdominal pain, deep rapid breathing, confusion or drowsiness occur. These are advanced symptoms of diabetic ketoacidosis. Failure to treat may lead to death.

Case-study 5.2 (Type 1 diabetes)

Miss Sarah Philips aged 24 years has Type 1 diabetes. She usually takes Actrapid 8 units and Insulatard 18 units in the morning and Actrapid 8 units and Insulatard 10 units in the evening. Sarah has vomited once and continues to feel sick. She also has diarrhoea. Her blood glucose readings range from 12 to 26 mmol/L and her urine contains small amounts of ketones.

Advice would include:

- Replace the usual CHO intake with fizzy drinks or fresh fruit juice. If unable to tolerate at least one glass to replace each meal, admission to hospital is necessary
- Perhaps contact GP and ask for an anti-emetic
- Test blood glucose and urine/blood for ketones four times a day. If blood glucose is less than 13 mmol/L continue with the usual insulin dose. If the blood glucose is 13 mmol/L or greater additional insulin is required at these times.

Suggested extra doses of insulin are:

- Blood glucose between 13 and 16.9, give 6 units of Actrapid insulin
- Blood glucose 17–19.9, give 8 units of Actrapid insulin
- Blood glucose 20 or above, give 10 units of Actrapid insulin
- If moderate/mid or large/high ketones are present and BG is 17 or above, give 10 units of Actrapid insulin

Therefore if blood glucose is 16.7 mmol/L at lunchtime, 6 units of Actrapid should be given. If blood glucose before evening meal is 17 mmol/L, 8 units of Actrapid should be added to the usual evening dose.

If blood glucose or symptoms are not improving or ketones worsen, urgent medical attention is necessary.

It is the role of the DSN and the diabetic clinic to ensure that those with diabetes are regularly updated in the management of intercurrent illness, particularly the adjustment of insulin. Gill and Redmond (1991) claim that the principles of self-adjustment to treatment are often poorly understood by patients. Unfortunately, people with Type 1 diabetes are still told by health care professionals to reduce or stop their insulin if they are ill, particularly if not eating normally. It is vital that every opportunity is taken to educate patients about the importance of continuing insulin and CHO replacement.

The use of large doses of oral steroids, for example in chronic asthma, will increase blood glucose. Management should be based on the guidelines above. If steroid therapy is frequently used it is vital that the patient is advised on how to increase his or her tablet or insulin regimes.

Those who usually require the maximum doses of oral hypoglycaemic agents may require conversion to insulin. Advice on how doses of insulin should be increased during steroid treatment is necessary. For those controlled on diet alone or on a small dose of oral hypoglycaemics, it is often possible for the patient to add extra tablets when required.

Travelling with Diabetes

Holidays are a disruption to 'normal' daily routine. It would be good if a holiday could be a holiday from diabetes too, but changes in diet, exercise and climate tend to make diabetes control more difficult and increased monitoring of glucose levels becomes necessary. Forward planning is necessary to ensure that diabetes does not adversely affect the holiday.

There is no reason why people with diabetes cannot travel anywhere in the world. It is advisable for those taking insulin to discuss travel plans with a DSN or a doctor if travelling abroad for the first time with diabetes. Advice will vary according to the needs of the individual. Before giving guidance it is vital to gain specific information from the traveller (Jornsay and Lorber, 1988). It should be established whether the person has Type 1 or type 2 diabetes (for further information please see p. 8). Those with Type 1 diabetes are prone to ketosis; detailed advice about what to do if ill, particularly with gastroenteritis, is therefore necessary. It is also more important to provide adequate insulin doses if the day becomes longer when travelling through time zones.

Diabetes control should be improved (if necessary) before going on holiday. The knowledge and experience both about travel and diabetes should be ascertained. For example, has travel sickness been a problem previously? Does the patient have any complications of diabetes, such as foot problems? Where the person is travelling to, and for how long; whether staying with family, in a hotel or alone in the jungle with no fridge will prove relevant to the advice required. The length of the journey, timings of meals and time zone changes require careful consideration.

General advice

Vaccinations

Travel to Asia or Africa usually involves a course of vaccinations. There are no contraindications for those with diabetes, although diabetes control may be temporarily affected. The BDA (now Diabetes UK) recommend that vaccinations be organized well before departure (1995b). The following organizations provide advice on the vaccinations necessary for various countries:

Thomas Cook Vaccination Centre
Tel: 020 7636 5553

British Airways
Travel Clinic
Tel: 0127 6685040

Further advice can be obtained from the individual's own GP or travel agent.

Some countries do offer a reciprocal health care agreement with the UK, providing free or reduced-cost emergency medical treatment. When travelling to countries of the European Union, production of an E111 form, which can be obtained from the local social security office or a main post office, entitles the holder to free emergency health care (Gill, 1992). The DoH leaflet T6, *Health Advice for Travellers*, may be useful.

It is advisable to take out travel insurance which includes medical cover; the minimum premium cover should be £500000 for holidays in Europe and £1,000,000 for elsewhere in the world (Diabetes UK, 2001). Diabetes should be declared and the small print on the proposal checked to ensure that diabetes is not specifically excluded from cover. Diabetes UK provide financial services which include travel insurance. Their Travel Quote Line can be contacted by telephone on 0800 7317431, Monday to Friday 8 am to 10 pm.

Identification

It is advisable for people with diabetes to carry some form of identification. Identification cards can be obtained from DSNs, diabetic clinics or from general practices free of charge, courtesy of diabetes product companies, or for a small fee direct from Diabetes UK. Identity bracelets or necklaces are available from jewellers or directly from manufacturers; for example:

Medic Alert Foundation
Tel: 020 7833 3034

SOS Talisman
Tel: 020 8554 5579

Many people with diabetes have found it helpful to carry a letter confirming that they have diabetes, their treatment, and a list of supplies that they will be carrying. These can be obtained from their DSN or doctor. Such a letter is particularly advisable for those carrying syringes in their luggage, although it is not compulsory.

Supplies

It is a good idea to take twice as much insulin/oral medication and testing equipment as would usually be required (Redmond, 1992). If travelling with a companion, supplies can be divided in case of loss. If the unthinkable happens and supplies are lost, most types of insulin used in the UK are available abroad although they may have different names. It is important for those on insulin to understand the action of their insulin so that alternatives can be obtained, e.g. if on 30/70 mixture to know that 30 per cent is soluble and 70 per cent is isophane insulin. Alternatively, the manufacturer of the patient's current insulin can be contacted before departure to ascertain whether it is available in the country being visited and the name under which it is manufactured.

Some countries use 40 and 80 units per ml strength insulin rather than 100 units per ml. Diabetes UK have a list of countries currently using U40 or U80. This list is, however, constantly changing as more countries change to U100. If 40U or 80U per ml strength insulin is used it is necessary to use 40U or 80U per ml syringes.

Long trips

A GP in the UK can prescribe a three-month supply of insulin (Steel, 1991) and testing equipment, which is enough to cover most holidays. It may also be possible to obtain further supplies from the diabetes clinic. If going abroad for longer periods it should be possible to obtain an equivalent type of insulin in most countries. A local chemist may be happy to send insulin abroad; if not, Diabetes UK has lists of chemists who are prepared to do so (Sonsken et al., 1992).

Storage of insulin

Storage of insulin whilst on holiday is one of the most common concerns. If travelling by plane insulin should be transported in hand luggage and not in the luggage hold. At high altitudes the unpressurized cargo hold reaches freezing point making insulin inactive and causing blood testing strips to under-read (Siddons, 1994).

Insulin manufacturers guarantee the stability of insulin at room temperature (up to 25°C) for a period of four weeks. Insulin should not be exposed to direct sunlight or extremes of temperature, for example in a car during hot weather. If

Table 5.2: Holiday supplies checklist

- Insulin/oral hypoglycaemic agents
- Other medication
- Blood/urine glucose testing kit
- Urine/blood ketone testing strips (Type 1 diabetes)
- Needle clipper and disposal container
- ID card
- Customs letter
- Carbohydrate-containing foods
- Glucose tablets/Lucozade, Coca Cola, fruit juice/Hypostop/Glucagon
- Artificial sweeteners
- Basic first-aid kit, e.g. dressings
- Anti-diarrhoeal medication
- Dioralyte

a fridge is unavailable insulin should be kept in the coolest part of the room, wrapped in a wet facecloth or placed in a wide-necked vacuum flask which has been kept cool.

Steel (1991) claims that insulin can be kept at 25°C for several months with a loss of only 2 per cent of biological potency; if kept for 10 months at this temperature potency is reduced by 5 per cent. At 40°C for several weeks, potency is decreased by 5 per cent. She claims that even in hot Third World countries without electricity insulin retains adequate activity for six months.

Soluble insulin should be discarded if it looks cloudy, and longer-acting or pre-mixed insulins should be discarded if they take on an uneven cloudiness or clumps remain after shaking (BDA, 1995b).

Diet

When travelling, dextrose tablets or other rapidly absorbed carbohydrate and additional and slow-acting starchy foods such as fruit or wholemeal biscuits should be carried if on sulphonylureas or insulin. Planes, trains and boats can be delayed, resulting in delayed meals.

There is debate about whether airlines should be informed of diabetes. Some airlines understand the modern treatment of diabetes and provide enough CHO (Redmond, 1992), others may not. Meals served may be low in CHO; extra CHO may therefore be needed. If airline attendants are informed, it is likely that those with diabetes will receive their meals earlier than the other passengers, which some have found beneficial.

Diets in Britain have generally become more influenced by other cultures and those with diabetes should no longer be on diets which are too strict and inflexible. It is helpful for the traveller to check on the basic form of the CHO eaten in the country to be visited and learn to judge the amounts necessary. A dietitian will be able to give specific advice if necessary.

In Britain and North America diet drinks are easily obtained but in other parts of the world this may prove problematical. Unsweetened orange juice is high in natural sugar and is unsuitable in large quantities. Low-calorie squashes may need to be packed if bottled or soda water or tea and coffee are not enjoyed.

Overeating whilst on holiday is common. If food intake is increased and exercise decreased an increase in treatment may be necessary. If symptoms of hyperglycaemia occur, those with diabetes can be taught how to self-adjust doses within safe guidelines before departure. Care is needed if alcohol intake increases.

Alcohol

Alcohol inhibits gluconeogenesis, thus increasing the risk of hypoglycaemia (Macleod, 1991). If sulphonylureas or insulin is being taken the negative feedback mechanisms which usually suppress endogenous insulin secretion during hypoglycaemia fail. This leads to a lack of available glucose in the bloodstream, which can result in hypoglycaemia that can occur several hours later (Appleton and Jerreat, 1995). Adequate CHO intake should be ensured; alcohol should never be taken on an empty stomach. Excessive alcohol intake should be discouraged; if more than three units of alcohol are taken at one time CHO intake must be increased. Low CHO beers tend to be high in alcohol and should be avoided.

Climate

Extremes of temperature affect diabetes.

Heat

Insulin absorption occurs more rapidly, which may lead to a rapid decrease in blood glucose. Those with neuropathy are at increased risk of sunburn. If the person is hyperglycaemic, dehydration may occur more quickly and cramps may occur. Large volumes of sugar-free fluids are necessary (Hillson, 1989).

Walking on hot sand may burn neuropathic feet; beach shoes should be worn by those with neuropathy. Some blood testing strips may over-read in hot weather. Insulin may be heat damaged (see section about storage of insulin for further information).

Cold

The rate of insulin absorption is slower, but when the person warms up it may be absorbed suddenly (Steel, 1991). This may lead to erratic levels of blood glucose.

If shivering occurs, the energy expended may lead to a hypo. If hypoglycaemia does occur, thermoregulatory shivering is inhibited and hypothermia can occur rapidly (Hillson, 1983).

Those with peripheral vascular disease and/or neuropathy are at risk of frostbite. Warm footwear is therefore vital, and specific education should be given to those at risk. Cold weather may cause blood testing strips to under-read.

Activity

This may be more or less than usual. Lying on a beach all day and overeating will increase blood glucose levels and an increase in tablets or insulin may be necessary. A holiday with increased activity such as skiing will require tablet or insulin reduction and an increase in CHO.

Illness

Illness, particularly diarrhoea and vomiting, can have drastic effects on diabetes. If someone is prone to travel sickness, anti-sickness tablets should be taken before each journey. Dioralyte may be useful if diarrhoea is experienced to help correct electrolyte imbalance. Discussion about what to do if ill, particularly for Type 1 diabetics, and the provision of detailed written information are vital before departure. The golden rule is never stop insulin or oral medication. Even if not eating normally the doses of insulin may need to be increased. Increase monitoring (including ketones if the patient has Type 1 diabetes); maintain fluid intake with sugar-free drinks and if unable to eat maintain CHO intake with sugary drinks. If the person is unable to tolerate fizzy drinks urgent medical attention should be sought.

Time-zone changes

When travelling east to west the day is prolonged; similarly, when travelling in the opposite direction the day is shortened.

Gill and Redmond (1993) reviewed the advice given by physicians running diabetes clinics to insulin-treated diabetic patients crossing time zones. Advice varied enormously: 7 per cent was unhelpful and 14 per cent was likely to cause hypos; many regimes were excessively complicated; 13 per cent of doctors recommended a basal bolus regime (see p. 45). Gill and Redmond recommended simple individualized advice without aiming for over-zealous control during travel. They concluded that local arrival and departure times may fit in easily with usual injection times in Britain, necessitating little alteration in insulin doses.

Like Jones et al. (1994), I have found that this has not been the case for many patients. There are a number of options available which depend on the type of diabetes and the level of control. The regime chosen should allow for flight delays, be as simple as possible and be the one with which the traveller is most comfortable.

The longer day

For example, Florida is five hours behind British time. Arrival at 1 pm will be 6 pm British time. If the day is longer, more insulin will be required.

Insulin adjustment: the options available

(1) Type 2 insulin-treated patients on bd regime with good control:
- Usual doses am and pm, doses 8–12 hours apart.
- As those with insulin-treated diabetes produce insulin of their own there is little risk of diabetic ketoacidosis if hyperglycaemia occurs.
- If poorly controlled, one of the options given for those with Type 1 diabetes could be considered.

(2) Type 1 diabetes patients on bd free-mixing regime:
- (a) Usual am and pm doses 8–12 hours apart with an extra dose of soluble insulin later with an evening meal (Steel, 1991). The dose of the soluble insulin will be dependent on the usual insulin requirements and the size of the meal. Siddons (1994) claims that 4–6 units are usually sufficient.
- (b) This is the method most favoured by myself, although not exclusively used:
  (i) Split the usual 24-hour insulin requirement into four to give 6-hourly insulin requirements. A dose of soluble insulin every 6 hours or so with a meal.
  (ii) Jones et al. (1994) suggest taking 15–20 per cent of the daily dose as soluble insulin before each main meal. It is not clear why only 45–60 per cent of the usual insulin dose is given despite a longer day and less activity. The authors do, however, suggest changing to 25 per cent of the dose as soluble insulin 6-hourly during intercurrent illness.
- (c) Another solution is recommended by Sonsken et al. (1992). Usual am and pm insulin, and after arrival a small dose of long-acting insulin prior to a well-earned sleep.

(3) Type 1 diabetes patients
- (a) As recommended in 2(b). Rely exclusively on soluble insulin.
- (b) Leave as pre-meal soluble and give nocte isophane at usual British time, e.g. 10 pm in UK is 5 pm in Florida, and give an extra dose of soluble insulin if an extra meal is taken.

It is important that nocte isophane is not given any more frequently than every 24 hours. Hypoglycaemia may occur due to the cumulative effects of intermediate or long-acting insulin taken more frequently than every 24 hours (Jones et al., 1994).

The shorter day

The principles are the same, although less rather than more insulin is required.

(1) If on bd regime:
  • Either take usual insulin twice a day 8–12 hours apart or change to soluble insulin 6-hourly.
(2) If on basal bolus:
  • Take soluble insulin pre-meal (may need only two doses) and isophane at the usual time, or change to soluble insulin 6-hourly.

Exercise

Exercise has traditionally been recommended as an important part of diabetes treatment because of its hypoglycaemic effect, and it continues to be so. With planning and appropriate advice most forms of exercise can be safely undertaken by those with diabetes. It is not only the more obvious sport-type exercise which may require adjustments to diet and/or tablet or insulin doses. A number of 'unexplained' episodes of hypoglycaemia follow gardening, window cleaning, shopping, sex, etc., perhaps several hours after the exercise has ceased.

The effects of exercise on the body in those without diabetes

• Energy is initially obtained from the breakdown of muscle glycogen and later from circulating glucose and non-esterified fatty acids (NEFA) (Ahlborg et al., 1974).
• Muscle uptake of glucose may increase twentyfold due to increased blood flow and glucose delivery and to enhanced glucose transporter activity (Ahlborg et al., 1974).
• Hepatic glucose production (glyconeogenesis) usually increases. However, after 2–3 hours of strenuous exercise without food, hypoglycaemia may occur even in those without diabetes (Felig et al., 1982).
• If a large sugar load is given prior to exercise, hyperinsulinaemia will occur which may cause hypoglycaemia within 30 minutes of exercise (Koivisto et al., 1981).

The benefits of exercise for those with diabetes

• Muscle insulin sensitivity increases significantly after 4–6 weeks of intense physical training (Koivisto, 1991).
• Hepatic insulin sensitivity is increased. This leads to smaller insulin or oral hypoglycaemic drug requirements.
• Lipid profiles become less atherogenic, HDL cholesterol levels increase, serum triglyceride levels may decline and total cholesterol levels may stay the same or decline.
• Exercise strengthens the heart, promotes circulation and lowers blood pressure (Hunter, 1990; Bouchard and Despres, 1995).
• Exercise may help to control stress and aid relaxation (Hunter, 1990).

- Exercise can lead to psychological benefits. These may include an improved feeling of well-being, greater self-esteem and peer acceptance (Rowland et al., 1985; Hunter, 1990).
- Exercise may aid weight reduction (Bouchard and Despres, 1995).

The effects of exercise in those with Type 1 diabetes

The effects depend on a number of factors.

(1) the level of diabetic control;
(2) the type and dose of insulin injected prior to exercise;
(3) the site of insulin injections;
(4) the timing of the last injection and CHO prior to exercise;
(5) the duration and type of exercise.

Blood glucose levels can fall (this is the usual outcome), stay the same or increase.

(1) If the control of blood glucose is good, blood glucose levels are likely to fall. Hyperinsulinaemia leading to hypoglycaemia is therefore likely if normal amounts of insulin have been injected. In those without diabetes, insulin production falls during exercise.

The presence of insulin prevents an increase in hepatic glucose production and prevents the normal increase in lipid mobilization during exercise; fewer NEFA are therefore available as an energy source. Insulin also stimulates muscle uptake of glucose.

If blood glucose control is poor and hypoinsulinaemia is present, hepatic glucose production is increased and counter-regulatory hormones are produced in increased amounts in response to exercise. Muscular uptake of glucose is inhibited and blood glucose increases further. Lipids are mobilized and ketones are produced. Those with hypoinsulinaemia are therefore likely to experience hyperglycaemia and ketonuria after exercise.

(2) Short-acting insulin given a few hours before exercise may peak during exercise and the use of intermediate or long-acting insulin produces higher peripheral insulin levels than normal. Hypoglycaemia is therefore likely without changes in dose and/or CHO intake.

(3) The action of insulin may be speeded up if it is injected into an exercised limb. Insulin should therefore be injected into the abdomen or buttocks rather than a limb prior to exercise.

(4) Ideally exercise should be started 1–2 hours after a meal (Koivisto, 1991). If a longer amount of time has elapsed between CHO intake and exercise, larger snacks will be required during exercise to prevent hypoglycaemia. Strenuous exercise should be avoided during the times of peak insulin action.

(5) During prolonged or strenuous exercise the amount of carbohydrate required per hour may be double that required during less strenuous

activity. In addition to increased carbohydrate intake, Sane et al. (1988) suggest that the insulin dose should be reduced by 40 per cent in strenuous exercise.

Advice

The advice given to those with Type 1 diabetes depends on their body weight, their level of understanding about insulin adjustment, the level of blood glucose control and the duration and type of exercise.

If exercise is unexpected, of short duration or occasional, an increase in CHO intake before and during exercise will usually prevent hypoglycaemia.

If the person is overweight, the exercise is going to be performed regularly, is of long duration, is particularly strenuous or hypos have previously occurred despite extra CHO, insulin adjustment will be necessary.

Food

The appropriate amount and type of CHO necessary varies. Koivisto (1991) advises 20 g of CHO before and at one-hourly intervals during exercise, some of which can be taken in liquid form. If exercising after a meal fewer snacks are necessary; larger snacks are needed if a meal has not been taken for two hours or more. Sane et al. (1988) claim that during strenuous long-term exercise a CHO intake of 40 g an hour with reduced insulin doses can maintain good blood glucose control.

CHO-containing meals and snacks *must not* be missed even if the blood glucose (BG) level is elevated after exercise. BG may fall many hours after exercise (even the next day) when the CHO stores in the liver and muscles are being replaced.

Testing

Blood glucose should be monitored before, during and after exercise. These results, together with insulin doses and CHO taken, should be documented to assess the effects of various forms of exercise and of the measures taken. Adaptations can then be made.

Insulin

The dose of clear insulin can be reduced before exercise by 30–50 per cent. If on a basal bolus regime this should pose no problems and dietary adjustment is usually unnecessary (Schiffrin and Parikh, 1985). If the exercise lasts for several hours extra CHO will need to be taken.

If taking a free-mixed regime, decreasing the morning clear insulin if exercising at any time after breakfast until lunchtime, or the evening soluble if exercising after dinner, is recommended. If exercise is taken at other times, or taking bd pre-mixed insulin, extra CHO will be required as reduction in isophane insulin is not immediately effective.

The effect of exercise in those with Type 2 diabetes

Peripheral glucose intake is increased in those with Type 2 during exercise but insulin secretion is decreased. Hypoglycaemia is therefore rare unless sulphonylureas are used.

Advice

Advice is dependent on body weight and the type of treatment used.

Those with Type 2 diabetes are unlikely to become hypoglycaemic if treated by diet alone, metformin or acarbose. It is therefore unnecessary to increase CHO intake.

If on sulphonylureas the dose may need to be reduced or withheld or CHO intake increased. The dose reduction necessary will depend on the usual level of BG control and the total daily dose usually required. If the exercise is of long duration or strenuous, unplanned, or longer-acting types of sulphonylureas are taken, e.g. glibenclamide, CHO intake should be increased.

Cautions

Certain types of exercise are more dangerous if insulin treated because of the risk of hypoglycaemia during the activity. These activities include scuba diving, motor racing, etc. However, with education and support people can often take part in some capacity. It is particularly advisable to have a companion if the activity is dangerous.

The advice of a doctor should be sought by the person with diabetes before an exercise programme is started, particularly if diabetic complications or other medical problems are experienced. There is an increased likelihood that those with Type 2 diabetes may have previously undetected cardiovascular disease.

Table 5.3: Possible cautions/contraindications to exercise

- Cardiovascular disease (particularly Type 2 diabetes)
- Peripheral neuropathy (risk of foot injury)
- Proliferative retinopathy (risk of haemorrhage)

General advice

- Hunter (1990) recommends a complete medical check from the consultant diabetologist or the GP before a strenuous programme is undertaken.
- Build up exercise gradually, e.g. by 10–15 minutes per day.
- Exercise at the same time each day to help with insulin/tablet and/or CHO adjustment (Hunter, 1990).
- Consider carefully the timing of exercise in relation to meal times.
- Shoes should be well fitting and comfortable. Check feet regularly for blisters or other damage

- Glucose tablets, Lucozade, Hypostop or other types of refined CHO should be carried at all times or be close to hand.
- Hydration should be maintained by drinking sugar-free fluids before, during and after exercise.
- The effects of the above should be closely monitored and blood glucose checked before, during and after exercise. Doses of insulin or tablets and amounts of CHO should be adjusted accordingly.

Reasons for avoiding exercise

- Lack of support (would like a friend to join them).
- Lack of time (work/family commitments).
- 'Not the sporty type' (lack perception of what constitutes exercise).
- Discomfort.
- Perception of appearance (e.g. in swimming costume).
- Media image of fitness (image that you must look superfit).
- Affluent lifestyles (cars, remote control TVs, car wash).
- Personal rewards (feet up after hard day).
- Lack of finance (e.g. swimming, gym).
- Fear of hypos/upsetting diabetes control (based on Smith, 1998).

Overcoming barriers to exercise

- Explore what personal barriers there are and discuss these.
- Define what we mean by 'exercise' – walking or dancing may be more acceptable than running.
- Use local exercise referral programmes as available. In Greenwich we have a Genesis programme which allows doctors to refer patients with medical conditions that can be improved by exercise. The local leisure centres then allow unlimited use of facilities at a greatly reduced cost to patients.
- Educate regarding adjustment of insulin/tablets and diet for exercise to prevent hypos.
- Start with small realistic goals – e.g. a 10 minute brisk walk for a previously inactive patient, increasing to 20–30 minutes daily over a period of 4 to 6 weeks. Setting small realistic goals helps to maximize feelings of success and encourages further increases in activity.

National Service Framework

The NSF standards relevant to this chapter are shown in Box 5.1. Standard 3 here should enable people with diabetes to travel, exercise, and so on. 'Minimizing the risk of recurrence' is important in standard 7; for example, cases of high blood glucose due to infection, or low blood glucose due to exercise.

Box 5.1: NSF Standards

Standard 3: Empowering people with diabetes

3. All children, young people and adults with diabetes will receive a service which encourages partnership in decision-making, supports them in managing their diabetes and helps them to adopt and maintain a healthy lifestyle. This will be reflected in an agreed and shared care plan in an appropriate format and language. Where appropriate, parents and carers should be fully engaged in this process.

Standard 7: Management of diabetic emergencies

7. The NHS will develop, implement and monitor agreed protocols for rapid and effective treatment of diabetic emergencies by appropriately trained health care professionals. Protocols will include the management of acute complications and procedures to minimize the risk of recurrence.

Questions (one for each learning outcome)

(1) *Illness*
   (a) Sidney has Type 2 diabetes. He takes gliclazide 80 mg bd. He usually tests his urine twice a week. He has a cough and cold and complains of thirst and passing large volumes of urine frequently. What advice would you give to Sidney?
   (b) Sian has Type 1 diabetes. She takes Humulin S (soluble insulin) three times a day, and Humulin I (isophane insulin) before bed. She feels sick although she has not vomited and she is unable to eat her usual food. Sian has performed no blood or urine tests because she feels ill. What would you advise?

(2) *Travel*
   Kathy has Type 1 diabetes and is travelling to Florida with her boyfriend. What advice would you give to her regarding storage of insulin, insulin adjustment and the supplies that she will need to carry?

(3) *Exercise*
   Peter and Andrea both have diabetes. Peter is 38 years of age and has Type 2 diabetes which is treated with metformin. Andrea is 29 years old and has Type 1 diabetes treated with bd Human Actrapid and Human Monotard. They are thinking of taking up badminton one evening a week and swimming on a Saturday morning. What advice would you give?

Suggested responses may be found on pp. 254–5.

References

Ahlborg G, Felig P, Hagenfeldt L, Hendler R, Wahren J (1974). Substrate turnover during prolonged exercise in man: splanchnic and leg metabolism of glucose free fatty acids and amino acids. Journal of Clinical Investigation 53: 1080–90.

Appleton M, Jerreat L (1995) Hypoglycaemia. Nursing Standard 10(5).

Bouchard C, Despres JP (1995) Physical activity and health: atherosclerotic, metabolic and hypertensive diseases. Research Quarterly for Exercise and Sport 66(4): 268–75.

British Diabetic Association (BDA) (1995a) Balance for Beginners. London: BDA, pp 51–2.

British Diabetic Association (BDA) (1995b) Make the break. In Balance for Beginners. London: BDA, pp 36–9.

Curry M, Weedon L (1993) Balancing act. Nursing Times 89(23): 50–2.

Diabetes UK (2001) Insurance and Diabetes Information Booklet, January 2001. London: Diabetes UK.

Felig P, Cherif A, Minagawai A, Wahran J (1982) Hypoglycaemia during prolonged exercise in normal man. New England Journal of Medicine 306: 895–900.

Gill G (1992) Diabetes, travel and holidays. Diabetes in General Practice Summer: 3–4.

Gill G, Redmond S (1991) Self-adjustment of insulin: an educational failure? Practical Diabetes 8(4): 142–3.

Gill GV, Redmond S (1993) Insulin treatment, time zones and air travel: a survey of current advice from British diabetic clinics. Diabetic Medicine 10: 764–7.

Hillson R (1983) Hypoglycaemia and hypothermia. Diabetes Care 6: 211.

Hillson R (1989) Travelling with diabetes. Practical Diabetes 6(4).

Hunter B (1990) The benefits of exercise. Nursing 14(6): 23–4.

Jones H, Platts J, Harvey JN, Child DF (1994) An effective insulin regime for long distance air travel. Practical Diabetes 11(4):157–8.

Jornsay D, Lorber D (1988) Diabetes and the traveller. Clinical Diabetes – a publication of The American Diabetes Association 6(3): 53–5.

Koivisto VA (1991) Exercise and diabetes. In Pickup JC, Williams G (Eds). Textbook of Diabetes. Oxford: Blackwell Scientific, Vol. 2, pp 795–802.

Koivisto VA, Karonon S-L, Nikkilä EA (1981) Carbohydrate ingestion before exercise: comparison of glucose, fructose and sweet placebo. Journal of Applied Physiology 51: 783–7.

Macleod A (1991) Employment, life insurance, smoking and alcohol. In Pickup J, Williams G (Eds) Textbook of Diabetes. Oxford: Blackwell Scientific.

Marsden P, Grant J (1991) Changing insulin regimes. Diabetes Care in General Practice Module 4: 1–14.

Redmond S (1992) Travelling with diabetes. Practice Nurse June: 104–5.

Rowland T, Swadba LA, Biggs DE, Burke E, Reiter EO (1985) Glycaemic control with physical training in insulin dependent diabetes mellitus. Sports Medicine 139: 307–10.

Sane T, Halve E, Pelkonen R, Koivisto VA (1988) The adjustment of diet and insulin dose during long-term endurance exercise in Type 1 (insulin dependent) diabetic men. Diabetologia 31: 35–40.

Schiffrin A, Parikh S (1985) Accommodating planned exercise in Type 1 diabetic patients on intensive treatment. Diabetes Care 8: 337–42.

Siddons H (1994) Travelling with diabetes. Practice Nurse March: 217–20.

Smith S (1998) Promoting exercise in Type 2 diabetic patients: how to achieve it. Journal of Diabetes Nursing 2(5): 155–8.

Sonsken P, Fox C, Judd S (1992) Diabetes at Your Fingertips. London: Class Publishing, pp 111–17.

Steel JM (1991) Travel and diabetes mellitus. In Pickup JC, Williams G (Eds) Textbook of Diabetes. Oxford: Blackwell Scientific, Vol. 2, pp 922–5.

Chapter 6
The care of diabetes in special groups of people

This chapter examines the care of diabetes in special groups of people. I have included the care of the elderly, ethnic minority groups, the pregnant and those undergoing surgery.

Learning Objectives

After reading this chapter you should be able to:

(1) Provide relevant, safe and specific care to elderly people with diabetes.
(2) Assess the information needs of, and provide appropriate education for, people from minority ethnic groups with diabetes.
(3) Give accurate advice and education with regard to diabetes and pregnancy to women with diabetes.
(4) Safely manage those with either Type 1 or Type 2 diabetes undergoing surgery.

The Elderly

Definition

There is no clear definition of 'elderly' or 'old age'. The dictionary unhelpfully defines elderly as 'somewhat old'. The term is generally applied to those of 65 years or greater. Whichever definition is adopted it is important to remember that there is great variation in terms of ability, capability and morbidity amongst those who are 'elderly'. Many people of between 65 and 75 years of age do not seem or consider themselves to be old and remain independent. Planning care for those who are elderly and have diabetes must therefore be undertaken on an individual basis.

Scale of diabetes in old age

Diabetes (both types but predominantly Type 2) becomes more common with increasing age. In elderly Caucasians the prevalence of diabetes is nearly 20 per cent and it is higher still in other ethnic groups (Meneilly and Tessier, 1995). Furthermore, the incidence of diabetes appears to be increasing (Stout, 1997). As the proportion of the population in western societies over the age of 65 is also increasing, diabetes is likely to be a growing problem in the future.

Why consider diabetes in the elderly as a special group?

Elderly people with diabetes differ from their younger counterparts (Sinclair, 1994). Elderly people tend to present with fewer of the typical symptoms of diabetes and may be asymptomatic at diagnosis. At least half of the cases of diabetes in the elderly are undiagnosed and diabetes is often present for several years prior to diagnosis (Harris et al., 1992). Established complications may be present at diagnosis.

There are some physiological reasons for these differences. The renal threshold for glucose increases with age. Glucose therefore does not spill over into the urine until blood glucose levels are higher, making polyuria less common in the elderly. Polydipsia is also less common because the recognition of thirst diminishes with age. Weight loss, if present, may be attributed to other factors rather than diabetes. If symptoms are experienced at diagnosis, the elderly person may present with confusion or urinary incontinence instead of classic symptoms.

Common problems in old age, such as immobility, multiple pathology, polypharmacy, problems with sight and hearing, poverty, social isolation and dementia all complicate the management of diabetes. Older people with diabetes have been shown to have greater knowledge deficits about their disease and are less likely to have received an education programme (Funnell, 1990).

Connell (1991) found that elderly diabetic patients had a higher frequency of chronic diseases and reported poorer health than age-matched controls without diabetes. Eighty per cent of those with diabetes felt that diabetes affected their quality of life and restricted their activities.

Chronic complications

The incidence of macrovascular and microvascular complications, peripheral and autonomic neuropathy and foot ulcers increases with age and the duration of the disease. Elderly patients with diabetes who are hypertensive, hyperlipidaemic, smoke or are physically inactive have a marked increase in the risk of macro- and microvascular complications. The prevalence of vascular complications and neuropathy is increased in the elderly who have poor glycaemic control (Meneilly and Tessier, 1995). This suggests that education programmes aimed at risk factor modification and attempts to improve diabetes control are worthwhile.

Caution is needed, however. There are no randomized controlled trials such as the DCCT or UKPDS which demonstrate the effectiveness of good control in reducing diabetic complications in the elderly.

Acute metabolic complications

Ketoacidosis is rare in the elderly (Stout, 1997). Its presentation and management do not differ significantly from those of younger people. Hyper-osmolar non-ketotic coma usually occurs in older people. The mortality of both conditions increases with age and exceeds 40 per cent in those over 50 years of age (Stout, 1997).

Cognitive function

Elderly patients with diabetes have a higher incidence of depression and poorer performance on a variety of cognitive tests than age-matched non-diabetic controls (Palinkas et al., 1991; Tun et al., 1990). Meneilly and Tessier (1995) claim that these changes are directly correlated with $HbA1_c$ levels, which suggests that improvements can be made. Meneilly et al. (1993) found that after six months of improved glycaemic control elderly patients had improvements in measures of affect, attention and concentration, retrieval of newly learned information and conceptual thinking.

Hypoglycaemia

Hypoglycaemia is the most serious complication associated with the treatment of diabetes in the elderly. The risk of severe or fatal hypoglycaemia associated with the use of oral hypoglycaemic drugs, and insulin is believed to increase with age. The elderly have reduced release of counter-regulatory hormones and reduced autonomic symptoms (Meneilly and Tessier, 1995) to warn of the onset of hypoglycaemia. Thomson et al. (1991) claim that elderly people also frequently lack knowledge of the symptoms of hypoglycaemia.

Many elderly people live alone, some may forget to eat and hypoglycaemia increases the risk of hypothermia. Strict glycaemic control is therefore rarely pursued, although individual circumstances need to be considered.

Management of the older person with diabetes

Sinclair and Barnett (1993) claim that diabetes care for the elderly is essentially unstructured, poorly co-ordinated, often inappropriate and in need of reorganization. Sinclair (1994) argues that this situation can be improved and makes a number of recommendations. These include district specifications for diabetes care, multidisciplinary audit, the establishment of screening and educational programmes, recognition of the contribution of spouses and other carers and the expansion of the role of geriatricians in diabetes care.

Watkinson (2001) suggests the appointment of a diabetes specialist nurse for older people. He or she could address the recommendations of the National Service Framework (NSF) for older people (Department of Health, 2001a), the national minimum standards for care homes (Department of Health, 2001b) and the BDA (now Diabetes UK) recommendations for diabetes care in residential homes (BDA, 1999) (see p. 157).

The aims of treatment

The whole person must be assessed and treated in the contexts of overall health, lifestyle, environment and wishes (Stout, 1997). Diabetes may be only one of a number of health problems with which the elderly person has to contend and it may or may not be a high individual priority. The elderly person and his or her carer (if appropriate) need to be involved in the decision-making.

The basic aims of diabetes care are to relieve symptoms and to prevent acute and chronic complications of the disease and its treatment.

It is obviously appropriate to relieve the symptoms of diabetes in the elderly. The issue of preventing or slowing down complications of diabetes is more contentious in those who develop diabetes in old age (Stout, 1997). With a limited life expectancy, microvascular symptoms may not have time to develop and macrovascular disease is commonly present in old age even in those without diabetes. The DCCT (see pp. 60–3) had an upper age limit of 39 years at entry. Its findings may therefore not apply to older people, in whom limited life expectancy and the risks of hypoglycaemia may make good control unnecessary or even unwise. Even the UKPDS (see pp. 63–5) had an upper age limit of 60 (median age 54 years), which again may make direct predictions based on its findings inaccurate for older people.

Diet

The diet is essentially the same as that of the general population (BDA,1992b). This includes regular meals, low sugar, low fat, high fibre and low salt and moderate amounts of alcohol. Although these guidelines are useful, modification may be needed. Factors such as age, weight, general health, cooking facilities, ability to get to the shops and financial status need to be considered. For example, an elderly underweight person with diabetes would not be advised a low-fat diet as their resultant calorie intake would be unlikely to be high enough to allow weight gain. A diet high in fibre may be too filling if appetite is poor and an increase in fibre intake should include a high fluid intake to prevent constipation. Coulston et al. (1990) argue that restricted diets may be an additional burden on patients who are dependent on others, and often make little difference to blood glucose levels.

Ideally, all patients should have a diet worked out specifically for them by a state-registered dietitian. This diet needs regular review and requires adaptation if circumstances change, for example if weight increases or decreases or treatment changes. In reality, a shortage of dietitians often makes regular review unlikely.

When discussing how to adapt recipes ounces not grams should be used.

Residential homes

Tong et al. (1994) looked at the process of annual medical review, and access to a chiropodist, an optician and a dietitian. They claim that elderly patients with diabetes in residential care received fewer services than those in their own homes when matched for age, sex and treatment type. Douek et al. (2001) found that only seven out of 33 nursing homes had diabetes management policies in their district. Nine homes stated that they would stop insulin in ill, insulin-dependent residents, and sharing of single use sampling equipment was commonplace. Reappraisal of the provision of health care in this group is needed, with specific guidelines and training.

The British Diabetic Association (BDA, 1997; now Diabetes UK) produced a free guide for residential nursing home managers and staff. This booklet includes advice on diet and alcohol, foot care, treatment, monitoring, hypos, sick day rules and the annual medical review. A 47-page report by the BDA in 1999 issued guidelines of practice for residents with diabetes in care homes. At the end of the report the working party stated that adequate funding for care within homes is needed and recommends the appointment of a diabetes specialist nurse and community dietitian to be responsible for care homes in a district. Sadly, this finding has not been implemented in many districts.

Oral hypoglycaemic agents

Oral hypoglycaemic agents should be used in the management of the elderly only when diet treatment has failed to reduce glycaemia adequately. The shorter acting sulphonylureas such as glipizide or tolbutamide are preferable in the elderly (glipizide is easier to swallow). It is generally recommended that longer acting drugs such as chlorpropamide and glibenclamide should be avoided in those over 60 years old, particularly when renal impairment is present.

Elderly patients are particularly susceptible to hypoglycaemia. An elderly person may forget meals and in practice it is often safer to take a tablet with a meal, so if the meal is forgotten the tablet is too. Tablet-dispensing containers may help elderly people to remember to take prescribed medication at the correct times.

Renal impairment prolongs the effects of some sulphonylureas as these drugs are excreted primarily through the kidneys. If the patient has renal failure either gliclazide or gliquidone or insulin therapy should be used.

Metformin is generally considered to be the drug of choice in the overweight patient. Metformin carries a risk of lactic acidosis in the presence of renal, hepatic or circulatory failure. Stout argues that it is perhaps better avoided in the elderly. However, Meneilly and Tessier (1995) argue that age has not been found to be a risk factor for lactic acidosis with the drug and that there has never been a reported case in an older patient with normal renal and hepatic function. Sinclair (1995) agrees that age should not be the primary barrier in the use of metformin. Stout (1997) accepts that it would be 'meddlesome' to replace treatment if an elderly person was well controlled on metformin or glibenclamide with no evidence of renal or hepatic problems or little evident risk of hypoglycaemia.

Few data are available on the use of acarbose in the elderly. Two small studies of short duration have been reported which demonstrated significant reductions in HbA1$_c$ and post-prandial glucose levels in elderly people with Type 2 diabetes (Meneilly and Tessier, 1995). The major side-effect of the drug is flatulence. This may be unacceptable to some elderly patients, particularly elderly women. It is advisable to start on a low dose and gradually increase. The drug has the advantage that it does not cause hypoglycaemia.

Insulin treatment

The elderly person with Type 1 diabetes obviously requires insulin treatment. Insulin may also be required by those with Type 2 diabetes.

Table 6.1: Indications for insulin treatment in the elderly person with Type 2 diabetes

- Symptomatic (particularly weight loss) despite maximum oral therapy
- Intercurrent illness/infection
- Painful neuropathy or amyotrophy
- Major surgery
- Hyperosmolar non-ketotic coma

There may be practical difficulties in the administration of insulin to elderly people particularly if they suffer from arthritis, impaired vision or dementia. Griffith and Yudkin (1989) argue that such difficulties may lead to poor diabetic control. It is vital to ensure that the dose can be administered safely. Can the dose be seen? Can the correct dose be drawn up? Will the patient remember to take it?

It is worth considering the use of pen devices, particularly the pre-loaded variety. However, some with arthritis find it hard to depress the plunger on pens. Pre-set syringes are useful, although it is possible to draw up air, the mechanism can slip and the dose cannot be varied without resetting the ratchet. A new pre-set disposable pen has recently been developed by Avantis; the Optiset. These methods cannot be used for free mixing.

Other patients use click-count syringes. These are of particular value if using a free-mixed regime, e.g. Actrapid and Insulatard or Humulin S and Humulin I. Many elderly patients may have been on a free-mixed regime for some years and may be reluctant to change their type of insulin. From 31 March 1998 click-count syringes ceased to be available from Hypoguard UK Ltd. This may have major implications for those using a free-mixed regime. Insulin regimes may need to be changed as click-count pens are broken.

Plastic magnifiers (BD: Becton Dickinson) are a useful adjunct to plastic syringes. They enlarge the figures on the side of the syringe and clip on to the bottle of insulin, keeping the bottle and syringe stable and making drawing up easier. Many patients who have arthritis or have suffered severe strokes can manage to draw up their insulin using this method.

Other options include a relative/friend/community nurse drawing up the insulin every 2–3 days and leaving it for the patient to inject; or a friend, relative or community nurse drawing up and giving the insulin.

Which type of insulin should be used?

Meneilly and Tessier (1995) claim that elderly patients make substantial errors when mixing insulins. Coscelli et al. (1992) argue that greater accuracy is achieved using pre-mixed insulin and that the level of control and frequency of hypoglycaemia were similar. I feel that each elderly person should be individually assessed and support given to enable him or her to use whichever type and method of insulin administration he or she prefers. As for all patients, this should be safe and as easy as possible.

Education

This should be relevant to the needs of the patient, simple and realistic. Before education is begun, an assessment of the needs of the patient should be made. Family and friends should be involved and information should be repeated as necessary. It is vital to ensure that the patient has heard and understood the advice. Opportunities should be given to practise handling equipment such as meters, pens or syringes on a number of occasions.

Of particular importance in the elderly is education about foot care. I have encountered appalling foot care by elderly patients. This includes the use of razor blades to trim hard skin and excise corns, pliers to cut toenails and the use of corn plasters and hot water bottles. Regular chiropody should be encouraged and arranged. 'Do it yourself' should be discouraged.

Information leaflets should be simple, relevant and in readable type size. Petterson et al. (1994) studied 15 leaflets routinely given to elderly patients in a diabetes unit: 10 per cent were found to be as hard to read as the *British Medical Journal*; 73 per cent failed to meet guidelines suggested by the Royal National Institute for the Blind which recommended 12 point as the minimum size for a readable typeface. Diabetes UK no longer produce a specific leaflet for the older person with diabetes.

Table 6.2: Guidelines for writing information leaflets for elderly persons

---

(1)   Use legible type size
(2)   Avoid unnecessary bold or italic type
(3)   Use short words and short sentences
(4)   Use illustrations which put across a specific message
(5)   Avoid unnecessary words
(6)   Be personal and avoid common use of the passive mood
(7)   Use concepts and phrases that all readers will understand
(8)   Avoid unnecessary capitals
(9)   Follow rules of grammar and syntax
(10) Obtain feedback
(11) Collaborate with skilled writers
(12) Pilot the leaflet
(13) Use first-generation photocopies

Source: Petterson et al. (1994)

Monitoring

This should be performed no more frequently than is strictly necessary (Stout, 1997). Urine testing for glucose has been considered unreliable in the elderly because of the increase in the renal threshold with age (Meneilly and Tessier, 1995; Stout, 1997), though Stout (1997) states that urinalysis may be adequate for those elderly people treated with diet or oral agents. In my experience urinalysis is often adequate if symptomatic control is the main aim of treatment. Home urine testing is easy to perform and the majority of elderly patients can do it independently, thus involving them in their diabetes management. We have described the use of a urine testing diary which has minimal writing, uses large print and requires only a tick to indicate the result (Weedon and Curry, 1994).

For those on insulin, blood glucose monitoring is necessary because of the increased risk of hypoglycaemia. Some elderly patients may be keen, motivated and capable of performing home blood glucose monitoring. For others, particularly those with poor vision, help from a relative, a community nurse, or the practice nurse may be necessary.

$HbA1_c$ estimations can be performed to indicate adequacy of control in addition to body weight estimation.

Screening/annual review

This may be undertaken by the GP, the hospital diabetic clinic, or the geriatric service. Multiple pathologies may lead to referrals to multiple clinics. Stout (1997) argues that one doctor should take overall charge of the patient's management; he argues that ideally this should be the GP, with hospital diabetes care reserved for specific diabetic problems. When there are several different clinical problems the Clinical Standards Advisory Group (1994) suggest that the geriatric service supported by the diabetes specialist nurse is most appropriate.

Minority Ethnic Groups

There are specific differences and difficulties experienced by those from minority ethnic groups with diabetes who live in Britain. Some of these will be addressed in this section.

Balarajan and Soni Raleigh (1993) have highlighted health inequalities which exist in ethnic minority groups in key Health of the Nation areas and in diabetes, infant death, haemoglobinopathies and access to health care. The Chief Medical Officer's report *On The State of Public Health 1991* (1992) argued that the NHS must address the particular needs of the black and ethnic minorities in England, be aware of ethnic differences and disease patterns and consider how these can be met by the provision of appropriate services.

In the UK the main research has been carried out on the Asian diabetic population (Marks, 1996). Samanta et al. (1991) studied diabetes in Indo-Asian and white patients in Leicester and found differences in the rate of diabetic complications, no educational materials in sub-continental languages and dietary advice inappropriate to the Indo-Asian culture. There was also no information available which evaluated whether treatment that worked in the white population actually worked in other populations. A lack of interest from national and local organizations was reported about the problems of the Indo-Asian population. Indo-Asian people were found to smoke less but to take less exercise than the white population. Morbidity is increased in the Asian population as Type 2 diabetes manifests at an earlier age and this is compounded by the fact that the population is younger than the white population (Marks, 1996).

Afro-Caribbean patients also present at an earlier age than Europeans. It is thought that the frequency of true Type 1 diabetes in the Afro-Caribbean population is much lower than in the white population (Odugheson et al., 1989). Treatment with insulin is, however, commonly required and Afro-Caribbean patients are more resistant to insulin, often requiring higher doses than white patients. They are prone to obesity and hypertension and may be predisposed to develop hyper-osmolar coma (Mather, 1991).

Type 2 diabetes is more common than Type 1 diabetes in all racial groups, but prevalence studies are not definitive. From the most reliable data available (Marks, 1996) mean prevalence, rounded up to the nearest whole number, is white 4 per cent, black 20 per cent, South Asian 25 per cent and Chinese 5 per cent.

Burden (1996) describes how diabetes progresses differently in the Indo-Asian and white populations. Twenty years after diagnosis of Type 2 diabetes most have progressed from diet treatment to tablet treatment to insulin treatment. Most Indo-Asians with Type 2 diabetes require insulin 10 years after diagnosis.

Gestational diabetes

Dornhorst et al. (1992) found that ethnic origin had a major influence on the prevalence of gestational diabetes. Compared with white women the relative risk of gestational diabetes is higher in all other ethnic groups.

Complications

Shaukat (1996) claims that Indo-Asians have increased prevalence, increased incidence, increased mortality and increased morbidity of coronary heart disease. Burden (1996) claims that when compared with white patients with diabetes, Indo-Asian patients with diabetes have less retinopathy and foot ulceration and more nephropathy.

The Afro-Caribbean population are at increased risk of stroke, renal disease and congestive cardiac failure, with ischaemic heart disease being less common than in whites (Cruickshank and Alleyne, 1987).

Treatment of diabetes

Govindji (1996) claims that the traditional Indo-Asian diet may change in the UK because of the switch to convenience foods, less time spent on food preparation and the greater availability of meats and cheeses. It may become higher in fat, higher in sugar and lower in fibre. The traditional Afro-Caribbean diet is generally high in starch and fibre but increasingly includes more meat and convenience foods. The Afro-Caribbean population is over-represented in the lower classes and is more likely to be unemployed; low income may affect food choices.

Govindji (1996) identifies fat in cooking, paratha and puris, gold top milk and fried snacks as the main sources of fat in the Indo-Asian diet. She recommends that Indo-Asian women be encouraged to measure cooking oil with a tablespoon rather than pouring directly from the bottle. The fat intake in the Afro-Caribbean diet is derived from fried foods such as dumplings and fritters, adding fat to food, e.g. jerk chicken, creamed coconut, hides and trotters, ackee and avocado pears and palm oil. This can be reduced by boiling, steaming, grilling and baking rather than frying. Low-fat spreads can be used and yogurt can be substituted for creamed coconut in some curries. Leaner cuts of meat should be encouraged and trotters and hides eaten less often (Govindji, 1992).

Like oil, salt may be poured directly from a large container; measurement with a teaspoon should be encouraged and, as with oil, advice given to gradually reduce intake. The Afro-Caribbean diet is often high in salt. Herbs and spices can be used to flavour food rather than salt, and salt fish can be soaked for a few hours to remove salt.

Lucozade and sugary colas are often thought to be 'health-giving' or needed for energy, and explanation is needed to indicate how the opposite is in fact true when the person has diabetes. Diet and low-calorie drinks should be encouraged. Sweetmeats are high in fat, sugar and calories, and gur is a type of unrefined brown sugar which, like brown sugar and honey, is considered healthy by some. Patients should be advised to eat sweetmeats only on special occasions and to avoid adding gur to curries and pickles, substituting artificial sweeteners.

Traditional vegetables such as karella have been shown to have a hypoglycaemic effect and should be encouraged in cooking. The juice from the ground vegetable is extremely bitter and is often taken as a medicine. If used in conjunction with oral hypoglycaemic agents/insulin it should be taken at regular times and the effect monitored to prevent hypoglycaemia. Guar (cluster bean) has been shown to lower cholesterol levels and should also be encouraged. High-fibre traditional Asian foods such as dahls and chapattis should be encouraged. Fresh fruit and vegetables are usually consumed at least daily. The traditional West Indian diet is high in fibre; peas, beans, lentils, yams, sweet potatoes and green banana are all good sources of fibre.

Extended families are common in the Indo-Asian population and the mother-in-law has considerable influence over the cooking and shopping. This needs to be taken into consideration when educating people of the younger generation or men.

Jones (1996) argues that the concept of 'food therapy' rather than diet may encourage the Indo-Asian patient to take it more seriously. It has been my experience that information will be taken most seriously if it is consistently given by all health care professionals. If GPs say one thing and dietitians or nurses another it is confusing. Govindji (1996) argues that Indo-Asian patients are most likely to see the doctor as a respected adviser.

Frost et al. (1992) claim that compliance with recommended dietary advice may be poor in the Afro-Caribbean population. They attribute this to the educators' lack of cultural awareness, the absence of specific written or verbal advice and the setting of unrealistic goals.

Diet or food therapy?

Jones (1996) advises that 'food therapy' alone should be tried for 8–12 weeks at diagnosis of Type 2 diabetes in Indo-Asian patients and that this is usually sufficient for a dramatic improvement in blood glucose levels. If tablets are required he suggests metformin or acarbose as first line rather than sulphonylureas, as insulin resistance is more marked in Indo-Asians. I have found tolerance of acarbose in Indo-Asian patients to be good, with less reported flatulence, although there are no studies to support this.

If insulin treatment is required in Indo-Asian patients the dose is likely to be higher: approximately twice as much insulin is required to achieve the same blood glucose control in Indo-Asians as compared with whites (Burden, 1996).

People from Indo-Asian groups are less likely to exercise. Samanta et al. (1991) found only 8 per cent of Indo-Asian compared with 33 per cent of white diabetics could be considered active. Exercise programmes which are culturally acceptable, e.g. Asian-women-only swimming sessions, should be encouraged.

Religion

Religious festivals and beliefs may have implications for diet and for the management of diabetes.

Indo-Asians usually belong to three main religions: Hinduism, Sikhism and Islam. Hindus do not eat beef and women may 'fast' one or two days a week although some fruits and milk may be allowed. The major Hindu festivals are Holi and Diwali at which an abundance of sweetmeats and other rich foods are available. The Sikh temple serves three free meals a day which include a dessert and a practising Sikh will usually attend for at least one meal a day.

Muslims celebrate the month of Ramadan, when no food or drink may be taken between sunrise and sunset. A heavy meal is usually consumed before sunrise and again on breaking the fast (Govindji, 1991). Ahmed (2000) argues that most Muslim doctors agree that Ramadan fasting is harmful for those with Type 1 diabetes. The religion itself exempts those with Type 1 diabetes from the fast. He suggests that liaison with a religious man may be necessary. However many with Type 1 diabetes do choose to observe the fast. Adjustments to insulin or oral hypoglycaemic agents may be necessary during this month if the person with diabetes chooses to participate. The insulin adjustment may simply involve the exchange of morning and evening insulin doses in those who are insulin treated rather than insulin dependent. It is against the Islamic religion to eat pork; it is therefore vital that pork insulin is not prescribed.

The majority of Afro-Caribbeans are Christians; a minority are Rastafarians and Seventh-day Adventists. As with the Indo-Asian population, religious beliefs may have implications for the dietary management of diabetes. Orthodox Rastafarians avoid processed and preserved foods, alcohol, salt, meat, fish, eggs, dairy products, grapes, raisins and wine. Seventh-day Adventists avoid pork and pork products, fish without scales and skins, and stimulants such as tea, coffee and alcohol.

Health beliefs

Before beginning to 'educate' the person with diabetes it is important to establish what they believe, understand and have experienced of the disease. This is important when educating anyone with diabetes; we all have our own individual ideas and beliefs. However, there are some beliefs which may be common within different ethnic groups.

Jones (1996) claims that there are a number of commonly held beliefs by people of Indo-Asian origin with diabetes. These include; 'If you get ill you either get better or die', 'If you take medication it will cure you', 'If you take the same tablets for a long time they build up in your body', 'If you have injections then you are very seriously ill'. Although the above may be more true of those of Indo-Asian origin, I have encountered many white people who share these sentiments!

I have found that Indo-Asians may be more fatalistic in their attitudes towards health care, believing that they have little influence on outcome. It is also common for the Indo-Asian person with diabetes to delegate responsibility to their wider family for monitoring of their diabetes, diet, cooking and even their exercise. It is therefore important to promote self-care and individual responsibility and decision-making.

Some Afro-Caribbean patients believe that God will heal them and I have met those who have stopped their insulin and/or oral hypoglycaemics in the belief that they have been healed or are in the process of being healed by God. Advice to these patients should be to continue blood/urine monitoring for glucose and ketones (if they have Type 1 diabetes) and to keep in touch with their DSN.

Obesity is considered socially acceptable as a sign of affluence in some Asian cultures. It is customary for guests to partake of hospitality foods which are usually high in sugar and fat content. Indian tea is traditionally made with evaporated or gold top milk and contains sugar (Burden et al., 1991). It is often made in a saucepan rather than a mug and it may therefore appear impolite to ask for it to be specially made or to refuse.

Education

A national survey of ethnic minorities attending diabetic clinics demonstrated poor provision of diabetic education aimed at specific groups (Goodwin et al., 1987). Hawthorne (1990) claimed that Asian diabetics knew less about glucose monitoring and complications than Caucasians. They had a negative attitude towards the diabetic clinic, feeling they were made to wait longer. They were also frustrated by the lack of communication with staff. Asians were found to have poor glycaemic control; despite receiving 'the same' education as 'British' diabetics, they did not understand it as well. The education was often seen as inappropriate and not relevant to their diet and customs.

The education of those from minority ethnic groups may be complicated. Patients may be unable to speak or understand oral or written English. There is a lack of educational resources available in languages other than English and which encompass different customs and health care beliefs. Ethnic minority groups do not form a homogeneous group. The Indian sub-continent alone has a population of over a billion who speak 1600 different languages (Jones, 1996). Even within groups sharing the same language, differences of class and religion exist. It is extremely important to base education on the individual needs of each patient.

According to the Health Education Authority (1994) only 32 per cent of Indians, 24 per cent of Pakistanis and 10 per cent of Bangladeshis living in England speak English. In younger age-groups English is now becoming the main spoken language but the incidence of diabetes does increase with age and language will continue to be a problem. English is read by 76 per cent of Indian people although this drops to 34 per cent of Indian women aged over 50 years; figures for the Pakistani and Bangladeshi communities are similar. English is read by 63 per cent of people from Pakistan but by only 29 per cent of men and 16 per cent of women over the age of 50 years. Of the Bangladeshi community 52 per cent read English decreasing to 38 per cent of men and 4 per cent of women over 50 years.

The majority of Indo-Asian people over the age of 50 years prefer to read non-English script. Illiteracy levels in the languages of origin are low. This strongly supports the need for educational material in preferred reading languages which include Gujerati (24 per cent), Punjabi (17 per cent), Hindi (2 per cent), Urdu (33 per cent) and Bengali (60 per cent). Languages most commonly read will depend on geographical area. Although some leaflets, in particular dietary ones, are produced by Diabetes UK and pharmaceutical companies, they are often not as 'glossy' or expensive looking as those in English, which I believe gives its own message to patients. Perhaps health care professionals should lobby Diabetes UK and pharmaceutical companies to produce all educational leaflets in a variety of languages. In particular, *Balance* magazine might adopt this approach. Leaflets specially aimed at various cultures and not merely translated from English would also be helpful. For example, as Asians are more prone to coronary heart disease and nephropathy, leaflets could be more heavily weighted towards these areas than towards footcare.

Videos and personal interviews by link workers have been shown to be most effective in presenting health education information about cervical smears to Asian women (Elliot and Fuller, 1991; McAvoy and Raza, 1991). Wilson et al. (1993) described a successful education programme specially for Asian patients in Asian languages using oral and visual teaching methods. The education programme was designed by an Asian link worker who was a qualified teacher and spoke many Asian languages, a diabetes specialist health visitor, and a dietitian. The link worker visited the homes of the patients the day before the education session and encouraged them to attend.

When teaching urine or blood testing for glucose to those unable to write in English a simple way of recording the results should be used (see p. 160). This will help support the patient's independence. Extra care needs to be taken to ensure that patients are aware of how monitoring will benefit them personally and not just the health care professional. Advice on how to contact DSNs is needed. We rely heavily on the interpreting service to take phone messages from non-English-speaking patients if there are problems.

Interpreters

The use of interpreters is essential if the patient does not speak English. Many hospitals and health centres now have access to an interpreting service. In the hospital where I work interpreters are available in all commonly spoken languages in the area. The two interpreters most commonly used in the diabetes centre have been trained by the DSNs in the areas of urine/blood testing for glucose, hypoglycaemia and basic dietary principles. They have also attended a diabetes conference as part of the diabetes team. They live locally and have contacts within the local community and temples and have taught us a lot about Indo-Asian culture and beliefs.

Burden et al. (1991) recommend the use of family members as interpreters if the patient has Type 2 diabetes. They argue that they have a high risk of developing the disease and are keenly placed to influence eating habits at home. This may be an advantage if the interpreter is in a position of power within the home, but is unlikely to be of benefit if she is the young uninfluential daughter-in-law.

Children should not be used, and the issue of confidentiality needs to be addressed if volunteers rather than hospital employees are used.

When an interpreter is used it is vital to speak to the patient and not to the interpreter. Extra time should be allocated when an interpreter is required. It is important that the interpreter relates exactly what you are saying and not his or her own opinion. A niece of an Urdu-speaking man proudly told me that she had added to the reasons for reducing sugar in the diet, 'if you don't stop eating sugar, the kidneys will fail, you will get gangrene and you will soon die'! Not the positive approach that most health care professionals would wish to employ.

The education and management of those with diabetes from ethnic minority groups can be both successful and enjoyable. Resourcefulness, sensitivity and a willingness to step into another's shoes when belief systems and attitudes differ from your own are, however, needed.

Diabetes UK produce some educational leaflets for those from ethnic groups; *Diabetes: A Guide for African-Caribbean People* (£2.00), *Diabetes: A Guide for Chinese People* (produced bilingually in Cantonese and English – price £2.00), and *Diabetes: A Guide for South Asian People* (produced in Bengali, Gujarati, Urdu, Hindi and Punjabi – price £2.00).

Box 6.1: Suggestions for a good diabetes service

The Audit Commission (2000) suggest that a good diabetes service for people from ethnic minority communities should:

- have information on the ethnic make-up of its population and target resources accordingly
- be aware of languages spoken, literacy rates, dietary practices, alternative remedies and religious practices
- have sought views on the services provided
- have appointed staff to reflect ethnic population
- train staff on religious and cultural aspects of diabetes care
- have accessible and 'used' interpreting service
- provide translations of literature and appropriate audio (and video) tapes
- have a policy for detection of diabetes
- give advice which is sensitive to cultural differences
- monitor outcomes by ethnic groups
- increase awareness of diabetes among high-risk groups.

Source: Audit Commission (2000: 38)

Pregnancy

Diabetes is the most common pre-existing medical condition complicating pregnancy in the United Kingdom, occurring in approximately four per thousand pregnancies (Brown et al., 1996).

Diabetes in pregnancy can cause numerous problems for both the mother and baby. However, the majority of women with diabetes can expect to become mothers of healthy children (Girling and Dornhorst, 1997). Despite this, many with diabetes have been given less than positive advice regarding pregnancy. This section will discuss why physiological problems occur, the risks to mother and baby, and the management of diabetes during pregnancy.

Changes occur in maternal metabolism during non-diabetic pregnancy. Girling and Dornhorst (1997) describe these changes as decreased fasting plasma glucose levels, increased post-prandial plasma glucose levels, increased fasting and post-prandial plasma insulin levels, beta cell hypertrophy and hyperplasia, decreased insulin sensitivity and enhanced lipolysis.

Metabolic changes in diabetic pregnancy

The decrease in insulin sensitivity means that those with Type 1 diabetes require increased insulin doses to maintain glycaemic control. Pregnancy-induced lipolysis also increases the risk of ketoacidosis in those with Type 1 diabetes.

Those with Type 2 diabetes already have decreased insulin sensitivity and the further demands pregnancy places on their compromised beta cell function usually lead to the need for insulin treatment during pregnancy.

Impaired glucose tolerance (IGT) may develop during pregnancy if women lack the beta cell reserves to keep blood glucose levels within the normal range.

Gestational diabetes/IGT

Gestational diabetes is glucose intolerance which is first discovered in pregnancy. Diabetes UK (2000) recommend the screening protocol set out in Table 6.3 in all pregnancies.

Table 6.3: Screening for gestational diabetes

(1) Test urine for glucose at every antenatal visit
(2) Laboratory test random blood glucose measurements:
    (a) Whenever glycosuria 1+ or more is detected
    (b) At booking visit and at 28 weeks gestation
(3) A 75g oral glucose tolerance test (OGTT) if the random blood glucose is:
    (a) > 6.1 mmol/L more than 2 hours after food
    (b) > 7 mmol/L within 2 hours of food

If the random glucose concentration is above 11 then the GTT should be omitted, the appropriate diet given and the need for insulin therapy assessed.

Gestational diabetes is indicated if the fasting plasma glucose is ≥ 6.1 mmol/L or venous plasma glucose is ≥ 7.8 mmol/L at 2 hours. Diabetes is indicated if the plasma glucose fasting is > 7 mmol/L and is > 11.1 mmol/L at 2 hours. Intensive treatment is required if the OGTT is > 9 mmol/L.

Since glucose tolerance changes with the duration of pregnancy, the stage of gestation at which the diagnosis is made should be taken into account. If diagnosis is made in the third trimester caution should be used, intensive treatment may be unnecessary.

Gestational diabetes usually develops in the late second or third trimester. Those with gestational diabetes should be cared for by the diabetic antenatal clinic, where dietary advice and advice on blood glucose monitoring with a meter will be given. Insulin may be required in 30 per cent of these patients (Thompson et al., 1994), though it will be stopped immediately post-delivery. Six weeks after the baby has been born an OGTT must be performed; if diabetes is diagnosed it is likely to be Type 2 rather than Type 1 diabetes. In most cases gestational diabetes resolves following delivery. There is a 30 per cent risk of developing diabetes (Henry and Beisher, 1991). This is more common in women from ethnic groups with a high prevalence of Type 2 diabetes, those with a strong family history of Type 2 diabetes, women who required insulin during pregnancy and those who are overweight.

Those with IGT or a normal GTT post-delivery should be advised on the importance of not becoming obese and of regular exercise. A random blood glucose should be measured by the GP every year.

Type 2 diabetes

The aims of care and management of those with Type 2 diabetes are similar to those with Type 1 diabetes. Tight control of blood glucose is required and therefore insulin is usually necessary. Ideally, oral hypoglycaemic agents should be stopped prior to pregnancy, and insulin substituted. Oral hypoglycaemics cross the placenta and are potentially teratogenic. Sulphonylureas stimulate fetal beta cells, which may aggravate fetal hyperinsulinaemia and macrosomia.

Type 1 diabetes

The aims of care include normoglycaemia prior to conception and during pregnancy and the prevention and management of diabetic complications. Advice about contraception and pregnancy should be given to every premenopausal woman routinely. Specific advice should be given in the hospital diabetic antenatal clinic to those planning to become pregnant. At this first visit a woman should have the opportunity to discuss the risks involved both to herself and her baby and how her pregnancy and delivery will be managed. Diabetic complication status should be established, folic acid supplementation advised, rubella immune status checked, advice about diet, alcohol intake, smoking and blood testing technique given as necessary and level of diabetes control established. If diabetes control is sub-optimal or complications such as retinopathy or hypertension require treatment it may be suggested that pregnancy is delayed.

Brown et al. (1996) argue that at the diabetic antenatal clinic a dietitian, diabetes specialist nurse (DSN), diabetes specialist midwife (DSM), physician and obstetrician should be present. They acknowledge that only 57 per cent of hospitals in the UK have a special diabetic antenatal clinic and in these clinics a DSM is available in only 25 per cent.

Before describing the specific management of diabetes in pregnancy I shall discuss the risks. I have made a rather unnatural distinction between risks to the baby and risks to the mother in a similar way to Fox and Pickering (1995) to illustrate them most clearly.

Risks to the baby when the mother has diabetes at conception

Congenital abnormality

Major congenital abnormalities are three to four times more likely to occur than in non-diabetic pregnancies. This risk is due to changes in blood glucose levels rather than genetic factors, as children of diabetic fathers do not share this increased risk (Girling and Dornhorst, 1997). High $HbA1_c$ levels are associated with congenital abnormality (Ylinen et al., 1984) and good glycaemic control has been shown to lower this risk (Steel, 1994). Kitzmiller et al. (1991) claim that the congenital malformation rate for those with poor glycaemic control who have not attended for pre-pregnancy counselling may be 12 per cent or more.

Most abnormalities occur between five to eight weeks from the last period, when many may not even realize that they are pregnant. Women are therefore advised to plan pregnancies and achieve good glycaemic control before becoming pregnant. Despite this, unplanned pregnancies with sub-optimal glycaemic control remain common. The Audit Commission (2000) found that one-third of centres visited did not offer pre-pregnancy counselling for women with diabetes.

The most common abnormalities affect the heart, central nervous system, the skeleton and face, the genito-urinary tract and the gastrointestinal tract (Girling and Dornhorst, 1997).

Spontaneous abortion / miscarriage

With good glycaemic control the risk of spontaneous abortion is no greater than in the general population (Fox and Pickering, 1995). Girling and Dornhorst (1997) claim that when poor glycaemic control leads to major foetal or placental abnormalities, miscarriage in the first trimester is likely but that no threshold of $HbA1_c$ concentration and rate of miscarriage has ever been established.

Large babies

Macrosomia is the term used to describe babies with a bloated plethoric appearance. Page et al. (1996) studied the effects of glycaemic control on macrosomia. Macrosomia was defined as a birth weight above the 90th centile using a computer model which took into account all the major determinants of birth weight. Twelve out of 29 babies were macrosomic. Fructosamine levels at booking were significantly higher in women who had macrosomic infants. The authors suggest that the incidence of macrosomia may be reduced by tighter control of diabetes at conception and in the first trimester but to a lesser extent during later pregnancy. This again emphasizes the importance of good glycaemic control prior to conception.

Maternal hyperglycaemia is only partially responsible for macrosomia; accelerated growth has been demonstrated in well-controlled diabetic pregnancies (Schwartz et al., 1994). More research is therefore required. Large-for-gestational-age babies are at increased risk of emergency Caesarean section, birth trauma, birth asphyxia, stillbirth and post-delivery hypoglycaemia (Girling and Dornhorst, 1997).

Stillbirth

The risk of stillbirth in diabetic pregnancies remains four times greater than in the non-diabetic population The exact cause of unexplained late stillbirths is unknown, although it is associated with poor maternal blood glucose control and foetal macrosomia (Girling and Dornhorst, 1997). Obstetricians are usually reluctant to allow gestation to advance beyond 39 weeks in diabetic pregnancies and will certainly wish to induce delivery at term (Fox and Pickering, 1995).

Hypoglycaemia

Approximately 50 per cent of newborn babies of diabetic mothers are hyperinsulinaemic at birth with beta cell hyperplasia (Girling and Dornhorst, 1997). After delivery the baby is unable to scale down insulin release when suddenly deprived of a high glucose intake via the placenta.

Small for dates

Small-for-dates babies are usually the result of maternal diabetic complications and generalized atheroma (Fox and Pickering, 1995). Placental blood supply is poor and foetal nutrition is therefore affected.

Maternal ketoacidosis

Fox and Pickering (1995) cite the foetal mortality rate resulting from maternal ketoacidosis as around 50 per cent. Kilvert et al. (1993) studied ketoacidosis in a combined antenatal diabetic clinic in 635 insulin-treated diabetic pregnancies between 1971 and 1990. A total of 11 episodes occurred (1.73 per cent); the overall foetal loss was found to be 22 per cent with only one foetal death in the seven episodes of ketoacidosis occurring in the second and third trimesters. Kilvert et al. (1993) argue that ketoacidosis is an infrequent occurrence in diabetic pregnancy managed in a combined clinic and that it is not associated with high feotal loss after the first trimester.

Respiratory distress syndrome (RDS)

The incidence of RDS fell from 27 per cent in the 1960s to 2.4 per cent in the 1980s, which is consistent with the fall in elective premature delivery and overall improvements in diabetic control (Girling and Dornhorst, 1997).

Diabetes

Inheritance of Type 2 diabetes is more likely than inheritance of Type 1 diabetes. The risk of a child developing Type 1 diabetes is about 6 per cent if the father has Type 1 diabetes, 1 per cent if the mother has Type 1 diabetes and 30 per cent if both parents have the disease. The risk of a child developing Type 2 diabetes is about 15 per cent if one parent has the disease and about 75 per cent if both are affected. If the mother or father has maturity-onset diabetes of the young (MODY) there is a 50 per cent chance of developing the disease (Leslie, 1991).

Risks to the mother

Nausea/sickness

This is a common problem in early pregnancy and is a particular problem in Type 1 diabetes. Insulin should not be withheld even if the usual food intake cannot be managed. Carbohydrate should be replaced in liquid form in the same way as during illness (see Chapter 5). Repeated vomiting can lead to ketoacidosis and anti-emetics may be required to prevent ketone formation. If moderate or large amounts of ketones appear in the urine, or liquid carbohydrate cannot be tolerated, admission to hospital will be necessary.

Hypoglycaemia

Achieving normoglycaemia during pregnancy increases the risk of hypos. Good control has been shown to increase the risk of severe hypoglycaemia (DCCT) and may influence the ability to recognize early symptoms of hypoglycaemia. Maternal hypoglycaemia does not harm the foetus but is disruptive and may be frightening for the woman with diabetes and her friends and relatives. Hypoglycaemia may be dangerous if driving.

The British Diabetic Association (BDA, 1992a) in *Driving and Diabetes* recommends that people on insulin who are unable to recognize early symptoms of hypoglycaemia should not drive. Dunlop et al. (1997) have found that 20 per cent of DSNs do not routinely discuss driving during pregnancy with patients and that over 80 per cent fail to advise women with unawareness of hypoglycaemia not to drive.

Steel (1988–89) argues that there appears to be a pattern to hypos in pregnancy. They tend to occur (1) in very early pregnancy up to about 16 weeks; (2) in the last few weeks of pregnancy, usually during the night; (3) around the time of delivery, during labour or immediately after delivery.

The DSN should be able to advise on the best ways to help to prevent hypoglycaemia and minimize the effects.

Diabetic complications

Prior to conception women should be assessed with regard to complications, diet and glycaemic control.

Nephropathy

There is no evidence to suggest that pregnancy accelerates a permanent decline in renal function (Fox and Pickering, 1995; Girling and Dornhorst, 1997). Davison and Lindheimer (1993) suggest that pregnancy is likely to have a successful outcome if serum creatinine levels are below 175 μmol/L and diastolic blood pressure is less than 90 mmHg before conception. When creatinine exceeds 250 μmol/L fewer than 50 per cent of the pregnancies have a successful outcome.

Table 6.4: Some common tips to reduce hypoglycaemia

- Frequent (at least four) blood glucose measurements a day with reduction in insulin doses and increase in carbohydrate intake as appropriate. If the blood glucose is low it should be treated with glucose and the insulin dose adjusted even in the absence of symptoms
- Regular meals and snacks should be taken and liquid carbohydrate given to replace meals if unable to eat normally. All patients should be seen by a dietitian
- Educate friends and relatives about how to recognize and treat hypos, to include the use of Hypostop and glucagon (see p. 121). Hypostop and glucagon should be routinely issued to all patients on insulin
- If night-time hypos become a problem it may be useful to 'split' the evening dose of insulin if on a bd free-mixing regime. Rather than giving both the clear and cloudy insulins before the evening meal, the clear should be given before the evening meal and the cloudy before bed. This delays the peak action of the cloudy insulin until around breakfast time
- If afternoon naps are taken, alarm clocks or phone calls from friends should be used to prevent sleeping through meal or snack times
- Before driving check blood glucose level, never travel when a meal is due and carry glucose. Driving should be avoided if hypos are frequent or if awareness of hypoglycaemic symptoms is lost

Hypertension requires treatment with non-teratogenic agents such as methyldopa. As pregnancy progresses the degree of proteinuria tends to increase and oedema may be a problem (Fox and Pickering, 1995).

Retinopathy

Fundoscopy should be performed and visual acuity checked before conception. Those with proliferative retinopathy require urgent referral to an ophthalmologist and pregnancy should be deferred until after treatment (Gorling and Dornhorst, 1997). Retinopathy may deteriorate rapidly if glycaemic control is improved suddenly and damage can sometimes be irreversible. Glycaemic control should therefore be gradually improved prior to conception in those with retinopathy. Hypertension during pregnancy is also associated with progression of retinopathy; good blood pressure control is therefore important.

Laser photocoagulation can be safely used during pregnancy.

Pre-eclampsia

The frequency of pre-eclampsia is 10 per cent in diabetic pregnancy compared with 4 per cent in non-diabetic pregnancy. This increases to 30 per cent in the presence of vascular disease (Garner et al., 1990). Women with nephropathy or hypertension pre-pregnancy are at increased risk.

Maternal mortality

Maternal mortality rate in non-diabetic pregnancies is 0.001 per cent (Chief Medical Officer, 1994) compared with 0.1 per cent (Cousins, 1987) in women with diabetes. It is highest in those with established microvascular and macrovascular complications.

Increased Caesarean section rate

Fox and Pickering (1995) estimate the section rate to be 10–15 per cent in non-diabetic pregnancies and 50 per cent in those with diabetes. A UK questionnaire showed the average rate of Caesarean sections in those with diabetes to be 44 per cent. The range between centres was enormous: 10 to 85 per cent (Brown et al., 1996). Brown et al. (1996) argue that in many units (44 per cent) women with diabetes are being induced needlessly early, which may explain the high section rate.

Management of diabetes during pregnancy

During pregnancy patients should be seen every two weeks and normoglycaemia maintained (blood glucose measurements between 4 and 7 mmol/L, HbA1$_c$ within normal range). HbA1$_c$ or fructososamine should be measured monthly. Fundi should be checked monthly and blood pressure, weight, urine and random blood glucose measured at each attendance. Dietary advice should be given at the first visit (ideally pre-pregnancy) and follow-up arranged as necessary. A meter to assess blood glucose levels should be lent to the patient if she does not already have one, and she should be advised to perform measurements at least four times a day to include some post-prandial readings. Serum creatinine should be measured and persisting albuminuria quantified. Weight gain should not exceed 10 kg (Marsden, 1997).

Diet

Advice should be given on an individual basis and must be affordable, acceptable and appropriate to religious, cultural and health beliefs (Brown, 1997). As for the non-pregnant woman with diabetes, diet should be high in complex carbohydrate and soluble fibre and low in saturated fats (BDA, 1992a); 50 per cent of energy should be obtained from carbohydrate. Women are advised to take folic acid 0.4 mg daily for a month pre-conception and for the first 12 weeks of pregnancy to reduce the risks of neural tube defects. This is particularly important for women with diabetes because they are at increased risk of these defects.

Education by DSN

An opportunity for assessment and revision of blood glucose technique arises when a meter is lent during pregnancy. There are many opportunities for discussion as patients are seen every two weeks. Insulin injection technique and dose can be discussed and patients taught how to self-adjust insulin according to home blood glucose readings. Women should be asked about hypos at each appointment and advice given about driving. Sick day rule advice should be given and phone contact numbers exchanged.

Once pregnant the majority of women with diabetes are well motivated and management becomes medically led following rigid protocols, i.e. visits every two weeks, HbA1$_c$ every month, intravenous drip during labour, etc. There is usually little room or need for negotiation. Although the DSN does have an important role as discussed earlier, I believe that the role of the DSN is most vital pre-pregnancy where the skills of listening, negotiation and compromise are most useful.

A useful booklet for patients is *Pregnancy and Diabetes*. It is produced by Diabetes UK and costs £3.00.

Ultrasound

- First trimester: crown–rump length should be measured to confirm dates.
- 16 weeks: provides further information about dates and excludes major congenital abnormalities.
- 18–22 weeks: anomaly ultrasound.
- Regular measurements of foetal head and abdominal circumference to assess growth should be performed every four weeks, and every two weeks during the third trimester. Weekly foetal measurements should be performed from 36 weeks until delivery (Brown et al., 1996).

Management of diabetes during labour

Brown et al. (1996) maintain that with good control and in the absence of significant obstetric complications it should be possible to prolong a diabetic pregnancy to 39 weeks and achieve a vaginal delivery.

Blood glucose during labour should be maintained between 4 and 7 mmol/L and blood glucose measured by the patient, her partner, or the midwife hourly. Intravenous insulin and 10 per cent dextrose should be given using a pump and a three-way tap to allow separate insulin infusion; 10 per cent dextrose should be administered at a constant rate of 100 ml/10g per hour (Brown et al., 1996). Marsden (1997) recommends that this should be increased to 120 ml/hr if ketones are present and reduced to 60 ml/hr for Caesarean section.

According to the protocol at Queen Elizabeth Healthcare Trust the insulin sliding scale rate should be calculated as follows:

(1) Calculate the patient's total dose of insulin per day prior to labour.
(2) Divide this by 24 and adjust to the nearest whole number (often 2) to provide the units per hour. This basal rate will need to be adjusted if dexamethasone has been used to promote foetal lung maturity in premature labour.
(3) A sliding scale may then be set as follows (blood glucose [mmol/L]/insulin [units per hour]):

- BG   3.9 or less   0.5 units per hour
- 　　　　 4.0–6.9   basal rate of insulin
- 　　　　 7.0–9.9   1.5 times basal rate
- 　　　　 above 10   double insulin rate and call doctor from diabetes medical team.

Table 6.5 gives an example of a sliding scale for an individual who usually injects between 40 and 60 units of insulin a day.

Table 6.5: Sliding scale during labour

Blood glucose (mmol/L)	Insulin (units per hour)
3.9 or less	0.5
4.0–6.9	2
7.0–9.9	3
above 10	4

The protocol for the management of diabetes to include labour and post-delivery should be agreed by diabetic and obstetric teams and an easily identifiable copy should be available in the hospital notes and the patient's hand-held notes. It should also state what should happen post-pregnancy to each individual woman. Continuous foetal heart monitoring and foetal blood sampling should be available during labour (Brown et al., 1996).

The infusion should be taken down once the placenta is delivered unless the woman will be unable to eat at the next mealtime. The pre-pregnancy insulin dose should be commenced with the next meal. If insulin has been used during pregnancy in women with IGT, insulin may be discontinued and an OGTT arranged six weeks post-delivery. If insulin has been used in a patient with Type 2 diabetes who is usually treated on oral hypoglycaemic agents, subcutaneous insulin may be required if she is to breastfeed. If bottle feeding, the woman should return to her previous dose of oral hypoglycaemic agents.

Breast feeding should be encouraged. An additional 40–50g of carbohydrate is usually recommended (Whichelow and Dodderidge, 1983) but despite this, insulin doses may need to be decreased by about 25 per cent (Alban Davies et al., 1989).

Arrangements should be made for follow-up in the clinic approximately six weeks post-delivery. Phone contact with the DSN may be most convenient during the first few weeks.

Surgery

Surgery is a form of stress on the body. The resulting increase in stress hormones can lead to increases in blood glucose levels and ketosis in those with diabetes. Peri-operative starvation may also increase the risk of ketosis. The type and duration of surgery, and factors such as infection and the presence of diabetic complications, influence the degree of metabolic disturbance. Fasting states may lead to a fall in blood glucose levels, resulting in hypoglycaemia if excessive insulin or sulphonylurea treatment is prescribed.

Responsibility for the management of the person with diabetes undergoing surgery is often placed on inexperienced doctors (Hughes and Borsey, 1994) and nurses. It is therefore important that simple and safe protocols are in place which are understood by all staff (Gill, 1997).

Pre-operatively

Good blood glucose control is necessary prior to surgery. Hughes and Borsey (1994) suggest blood glucose levels between 6.7 and 10 mmol/L. For some with Type 2 diabetes this may mean conversion to insulin prior to surgery. It is important that fitness for surgery is confirmed. Pre-operative assessment should include routine biochemistry, urinalysis, ECG and chest X-ray (Hughes and Borsey, 1994). Fundoscopy should be performed if anti-coagulant therapy is likely to be used.

Those with peripheral neuropathy are at increased risk of pressure sores because of impaired sensation. This should be identified at medical and nursing assessment of the patient and competent pressure area care should be given. Gill (1997) states that close liaison between the diabetes care team, surgeons and anaesthetists is essential. Ideally surgery should be scheduled for the morning – first on the list if possible.

The patient should have the opportunity to ask questions and be given information not only about the nature of surgery but about the management of his or her diabetes. Some with diabetes may have heard horror stories, or even experienced problems with diabetes management as an inpatient. Reassurance that insulin will be given continuously if they are insulin dependent and that a dextrose infusion will prevent hypoglycaemia, is important. The patient may also need reassurance about the accuracy of nurses' blood glucose monitoring technique. Those on insulin have been used to taking responsibility for their own blood glucose control and may find it frightening to lose this control to others. Wherever possible a member of the diabetes team should be involved.

Management

Gill (1997) suggests that the blood glucose range should be maintained between 6 and 11 mmol/L. Lower blood glucose levels should be avoided because of the risk of hypoglycaemia. Hypos are particularly important to avoid as the patient may be unable to recognize hypos or be unable to communicate. Management is determined by the type of diabetes, i.e. whether the patient has Type 2 or Type 1 diabetes, the type and duration of the surgery, the level of diabetic control and the length of time that the patient will need to fast.

It is safest to assume that those treated with insulin have no insulin of their own and therefore will require a continuous supply of exogenous insulin. Those with Type 2 diabetes who are usually controlled on diet or diet and tablets will usually require insulin only if undergoing major surgery.

Management of patients treated by diet, or diet and tablets

Hughes and Borsey (1994) argue that all patients should be admitted to hospital two days before surgery for assessment of blood glucose control. However, in practice this may not always be possible. Therefore, if surgery is planned diabetes specialist nurses should ideally be involved at an early stage a number of weeks before admission to assess and if necessary improve diabetes control.

Tablets

Chlorpropamide should be stopped at least 5–7 days before surgery (Hughes and Borsey, 1994; Gill, 1997). A shorter-acting sulphonylurea such as glipizide, tolbutamide or gliclazide should be substituted to reduce the risk of hypoglycaemia during fasting. Metformin should also be stopped 5–7 days prior to surgery (Hughes and Borsey, 1994) because of the small risk of lactic acidosis.

Minor surgery

Tablets should be omitted on the morning of the operation. Blood glucose should be checked before and after surgery and tablets restarted with the first main meal. If the patient is poorly controlled, insulin should be used pre-, during or post-surgery. Glucose-containing infusions should be avoided when insulin is not infused.

Major surgery

Continuous glucose and insulin delivery should be used as for Type 1 diabetes patients.

Insulin-treated patients

Prior to and post-surgery urinalysis should be performed or blood test for ketones. If ketones occur when blood glucose is less than 10 mmol/L more dextrose is required; if blood glucose is greater than 10 mmol/L more insulin is necessary.

There are two methods commonly used to provide a continuous supply of glucose and insulin.

Method 1: The separate line system

This is the method favoured in the hospital in which I work and also by Hughes and Borsey (1994). This allows separate adjustment of the insulin and dextrose. The infusions can be given into separate veins or the insulin infusion can be piggy-backed into the glucose line. One infusion provides 10 per cent glucose and if infused at 100 ml per hour it will provide 10 g of glucose per hour, the recommended minimum. An electronic drip counter should be used whenever possible (Gill, 1997) to ensure continuous glucose supply. Soluble insulin (Actrapid, Humulin S, Velosulin) is placed in 0.9 per cent saline in a 50 ml syringe to provide 50 units of insulin in 50 ml of saline. The syringe driver pump can be set to provide insulin at 2–6 units per hour. Gill (1997) argues that 2–4 units per hour is the most usual dose. The rate can be calculated in a similar way to during labour – see Table 6.5 (p. 176). Blood glucose testing should be performed hourly, ideally with a meter by a nurse trained and competent in its use. The insulin infusion rate should start at 2 units per hour and be increased according to blood glucose readings. Serum potassium should be checked prior to and two hours post-surgery and KCl added to the dextrose infusion as necessary.

Method 2: The glucose potassium regime (GKI)

Husband et al. (1986) describe this method as simple and effective and it is the method favoured by Gill (1997).

In this regime, 15 units of soluble insulin and 5 mmol of potassium chloride are added to 500 ml of 10 per cent glucose. The mixture is infused at 100 ml per hour. The advantage of this method is that glucose and insulin are delivered simultaneously and a pump is therefore not essential. In method 1 there is a danger that if the glucose infusion finishes but the insulin continues, hypoglycaemia will occur. This potential problem can be overcome by using alarms (Hughes and Borsey, 1994).

The insulin and potassium doses should be added to the bag of dextrose using a needle which is long enough to bypass the bung. The bag requires to be mixed well and to be labelled clearly. Blood glucose monitoring should be performed at least hourly until insulin requirements are stable.

The insulin rate can be altered only by substituting a new bag containing a different dosage. Gill (1997) suggests that if blood glucose is greater than 11 mmol/L then the GKI contains 20 units; if blood glucose is less than 6 mmol/L then the GKI infusion contains 10 units of insulin. Gill (1997) claims that alterations in the standard GKI infusion are rarely needed.

Post-operatively

Whichever method is used, the drip can be discontinued when the patient resumes eating. Hughes and Borsey (1994) suggest that subcutaneous insulin be given one hour prior to the discontinuation of the insulin but make no suggestions regarding the dose. Gill (1997) suggests that the patient should revert to 'usual' treatment.

Our hospital protocol suggests substituting the drip with tds subcutaneous soluble insulin in a dose determined by need in cases of difficulty and warns against using a sliding scale, which can lead to wide fluctuations in blood glucose levels. Insulin needs should be determined by reference to the pre-operative total daily dose and the intravenous dose required during surgery. This protocol suggests a possible need for increase of dose for catabolism and infection.

In general, if the patient's insulin requirements during surgery have been similar to the normal daily requirements then the normal subcutaneous dosage should be given prior to the evening meal. If the dose requirements have been increased during surgery, soluble insulin should be given tds based on these requirements. For example, if the usual dose of insulin was Actrapid 8 units and Insulatard 22 units am and Actrapid 4 units and Insulatard 14 units pm (a total of 48 units) and an insulin infusion rate of 2 units per hour had maintained blood glucose between 7 and 10mmol/L, the usual type and dose of insulin could be given. If the rate required had varied and was usually greater than 2 units an hour then tds soluble insulin should be used.

If the patient is vomiting or feels unable to eat, the intravenous infusion should be continued.

Case-study 6.1

Winifred Smith has Type 1 diabetes and is to undergo a hysterectomy. Her usual insulin doses are Humulin S 10 units and Humulin I 20 units in the morning and Humulin S 6 units and Humulin I 14 units in the evening (thus requiring approximately 2 units of insulin an hour).

Suggested care would include:

Pre-op:

- Discussion with patient about how diabetes will be managed
- Ensure good blood glucose control
- Medical assessment
- Check serum potassium
- Ideally first on morning list.

Day of surgery:

- No subcutaneous insulin/breakfast
- Nil by mouth
- Test urine (or blood) for ketones
- Set up infusions:
  10 per cent dextrose at 100 ml/hour
  Soluble insulin 50 units in 50 ml 0.9 per cent saline
- Monitor blood glucose hourly
- Start insulin infusion at 2 units per hour
- Adjust rate of insulin according to scale indicated in Table 6.6.

Table 6.6:

Blood glucose (mmol/L)		Suggested insulin rate (ml/hr)
3.9 or less	0.5	
4.0–6.9	2	(basal rate of insulin)
7.0–9.9	3	(1.5 times basal rate)
10.0–16.9	4	double basal rate)
17.0 or above	6	(treble basal rate and call doctor)

Post-op:

- 1–2 hourly blood glucose measurements
- After two hours, serum potassium should be checked
- When the patient is eating, give subcutaneous dose of insulin $\frac{1}{2}$ hour before infusions are discontinued and meal is eaten
- When pump discontinued, six-hourly blood glucose measurements
- Test urine (or blood) for ketones.

Emergency surgery

The problem which makes emergency surgery necessary may have led to significant metabolic disturbance in the person with diabetes, particularly in those with Type 1 diabetes. It is important that the patient is fully assessed prior to surgery, including measurement of blood gases (Hughes and Borsey, 1994). If dehydration or acidosis are present, these should be corrected prior to surgery. Increased insulin infusion rates may be required.

Principles of treatment for outpatient investigations which require adjustment to food intake

Local protocols may be in place. In the hospital in which I work specific guidelines exist for those with diabetes undergoing barium meal, abdominal ultrasound, CT scan, intravenous urogram (IVU), gall bladder scan and examinations requiring bowel preparation with Picolax.

As with surgery, it is important to distinguish between those who are treated with insulin and those treated with diet and diet and tablets. There is a risk of ketosis in those with Type 1 diabetes if insulin is withheld. Those treated with sulphonylureas or insulin risk hypoglycaemia if food intake is reduced unless simple guidelines are followed.

The investigation should be scheduled for 9.30 am in those treated with insulin or tablets. If dietary restrictions are needed prior to the investigation, carbohydrate-containing foods, e.g. bread, potatoes, etc., should be replaced with liquid carbohydrate. On the morning of the investigation oral hypoglycaemics or insulin should be omitted if the patient is not allowed to eat or drink. The insulin or tablets, in addition to carbohydrate-containing food, can be given immediately the investigation is completed. Adjustments to insulin and tablet regimes may be necessary if the investigation is not completed by 11 am to prevent morning doses of hypoglycaemic agents overlapping with the evening doses (see Figure 6.1 for suggested protocol for CT scan and diabetes). Patients should be instructed to treat any hypoglycaemic episodes with dextrose tablets rather than liquid carbohydrate if 'nil by mouth'.

If X-ray contrast is required, such as in the cases of IVU and CT scans, metformin should be omitted on the day of, and for two days after the investigation. There is an increased risk of lactic acidosis (Royal College of Radiologists, 1998).

CT Body Scan

ADDITIONAL ADVICE FOR THOSE WITH DIABETES TREATED WITH INSULIN.

Ideally, the time of the appointment for your investigation should be early in the morning (9–9.30 am). However, as this is a very specialized investigation, sometimes it may be necessary for you to have an appointment at a later time. Please seek further advice if necessary from the Diabetes Centre.

ON THE DAY OF THE EXAMINATION (early morning appointment).

Do not take your usual insulin

Test your blood glucose on waking: if it is less than 4 mmol/L treat as hypo with dextrose tablets, **not** liquid carbohydrate.

Figure 6.1: Patient advice for CT scan and diabetes

Take insulin supplies, blood testing kit, dextrose tablets and a sandwich to the hospital with you.

If your blood glucose falls to below 4 mmol/L at any time, treat with dextrose tablets.

Immediately after the examination is finished take your usual dose of insulin and eat your sandwich. Then continue your day as usual.

If the examination has not finished by 11 am **do not take your usual insulin but proceed as follows:**

If you usually mix clear and cloudy insulin together in a syringe take clear insulin dose **only** before lunch and then continue with your usual insulin before the evening meal.

If you usually take a premixed insulin, e.g. Humulin M2, M3, or Mixtard, please ring the Diabetes Centre for advice on what to do.

If you take only one injection a day please ring the Diabetes Centre before the date of the examination and discuss what to do!

ADDITIONAL ADVICE FOR THOSE WITH DIABETES TREATED WITH TABLETS

If treated with metformin – this must be stopped on the day of the investigation. Please ring the Diabetes Centre immediately you receive the appointment. You will need further individual instructions.

As this is a very specialized investigation, sometimes it may be necessary for you to have an appointment at a time later than 9 am. Please seek further advice from the Diabetes Centre as necessary.

ON THE DAY OF THE EXAMINATION (early morning appointment).

Do **not** take your diabetic tablets prior to the examination.

If you experience symptoms of a low blood sugar (sweating, shaking, pins & needles sensations etc.) suck 3 glucose tablets. **Do not** take liquid carbohydrate (sugary drinks).

If your examination is completed by 11 am take your usual morning dose of tablets followed by breakfast.

If your examination is not completed by 11 am eat as usual but **do not** take your morning dose of tablets. Take your usual evening dose at the normal time (except if you take metformin).

If you usually only take a morning dose of your tablets, take your usual morning dose before your first main meal after your examination.

If you are treated with metformin tablets these must not be taken for 2 days after the investigation.

FOR APPOINTMENTS 11 AM OR LATER

It is important that you do not eat or drink anything for 4 hours before the scan. For a person with diabetes this could obviously be problematic.

If you are treated with diet alone

No additional instructions are needed. Please follow the instructions for those without diabetes.

Figure 6.1: Patient advice for CT scan and diabetes (contd)

If you are treated with metformin (Glucophage) alone

These should be stopped 2 days before the investigation and not taken for 2 days after the investigation. Please telephone the Diabetes Centre for individual advice.

If you are treated with tablets other than metformin (Glucophage) or acarbose (Glucobay)

If you are on chlorpropamide (Diabenese) tablets, these need to be changed to different tablets a week before the appointment and you should contact the Diabetes Centre as soon as possible.

Take your usual dose of gliclazide (Diamicron), glibenclamide (Daonil), glipizide (Glibenese), or repaglinide (NovoNorm), and have your breakfast as usual, which should be at least 4 hours before the scan.

For example, if your appointment is at 1 pm you can eat normally until 9 am – snacks and lunch will need to be replaced with another form of carbohydrate (see starch food exchange list).

If your appointment is at 4 pm you may eat until 12 noon. Snacks after this time will need to be replaced with items from the starch food exchange list.

There is a risk of low blood sugar because you may be unable to eat your normal amount of starchy foods. Because of this your usual amounts of starch have to be replaced by dextrose tablets or small amounts of fluid containing sugar if a snack or meal cannot be taken (see starch food exchange list).

For those treated with insulin

Take your usual dose of insulin in the morning and have your breakfast at your usual time, which should be at least 4 hours before the scan.

For example, if your appointment is at 1 pm you can eat normally until 9 am – snacks and lunch will need to be replaced with another form of carbohydrate (see starch food exchange list).

If your appointment is at 4 pm you may eat until 12 noon. Snacks after this time will need to be replaced with items from the starch food exchange list.

There is a risk of low blood sugar because you may be unable to eat your normal amount of starchy foods. Because of this your usual amounts of starch have to be replaced by dextrose tablets or small amounts of fluid containing sugar if a snack or meal cannot be taken (see starch food exchange list).

FOR APPOINTMENTS LATER THAN 5 PM

Please contact the Diabetes Centre prior to investigation for individual advice. Have lunch as usual, not later than 1 pm.

Snacks after this time should be replaced using items from the starch food exchange list.

The evening insulin dose should be given but may require adjustment, please contact the Diabetes Centre for individual advice. Carbohydrate foods and snacks will need replacement with items from starch exchange list.

Figure 6.1: (contd) Devised by Lynne Jerreat and Cathy Parker (1997) © DDCC. GDH

STARCH FOOD EXCHANGE LIST

The following provide approximately 1 portion of carbohydrate:

1 slice of bread

1 medium chapatti

1 medium potato

1 serving spoon of rice or pasta

1 digestive biscuit

1 bowl of breakfast cereal

1 packet of crisps

1 piece of fruit, e.g. a banana

1 yogurt

1 glass of milk

THESE CAN BE EXCHANGED FOR:

(Drinks must **not** be fizzy (this affects the investigation). Sugar can be added and the liquid stirred to remove the fizz)

1/4 glass (50 ml/2 fl oz) Lucozade with 1 teaspoon of sugar

1/2 glass (100 ml/4 fl oz) of **ordinary** coke with 1 teaspoon sugar

1 cup of black tea or coffee with 2 teaspoons of sugar

25 ml/1 fl oz undiluted Ribena made up to taste with water

Figure 6.1: (contd) Devised by Lynne Jerreat and Cathy Parker (1997) © DDCC. GDH

National Service Framework

The NSF Standards relevant to this chapter are shown in Box 6.2. Standard 2 should include screening pre-surgery, during pregnancy and for people over 75 years in high-risk groups. Standards 11 and 12 include surgery for complications of diabetes, such as eye treatment, amputation, and so on.

Box 6.2: NSF Standards (DoH, 2001c)

Standard 2: Identification of people with diabetes

(2)   The NHS will develop, implement and monitor strategies to identify people who do not know they have diabetes.

Standard 3: Empowering people with diabetes

(3)   All children, young people and adults with diabetes will receive a service which encourages partnership in decision-making, supports them in managing their diabetes and helps them to adopt and maintain a healthy lifestyle. This will be reflected in an agreed and shared care plan in an appropriate format and language. Where appropriate, parents and carers should be fully engaged in this process.

Standard 8: Care of people with diabetes during admission to hospital

(8)   All children, young people and adults with diabetes admitted to hospital, for whatever reason, will receive effective care of their diabetes. Whenever possible, they will continue to be involved in decisions concerning the management of their diabetes.

Standard 9: Diabetes and Pregnancy

(9)   The NHS will develop, implement and monitor policies that seek to empower and support women with pre-existing diabetes and those who develop diabetes during pregnancy to optimize the outcome of their pregnancy.

Standards 11 and 12: Management of long-term complications

(11)   The NHS will develop, implement and monitor agreed protocols and systems of care to ensure that all people who develop long-term complications of diabetes receive timely, appropriate and effective investigation and treatment to reduce their risk of disability and premature death.
(12)   All people with diabetes requiring multi-agency support will receive integrated health and social care.

Questions (one for each learning outcome)

(1) Mr Alexander is 92 years of age and has had Type 2 diabetes for 30 years. He takes gliclazide 160 mg bd and metformin 500 mg tds. Mr Alexander complains of getting up to pass urine at least four times during the night, thirst, lack of energy and weight loss of about one and a half stones over the last six months. He believes these symptoms to be due to the fact that he is getting old. Do you think Mr Alexander's treatment needs changing? If so, to what? What factors will need to be taken into consideration?

(2) Mrs Patel has newly diagnosed Type 2 diabetes. She speaks Punjabi and understands a limited amount of English. Mrs Patel needs education and advice about how to control and monitor her diabetes. What further information do you need? What advice and treatment do you feel to be needed initially?

(3) Helen Palmer is 30 years old and has had Type 1 diabetes for 15 years. She is keen to start a family but comments made to her by a health care professional when she was a teenager were not encouraging. What advice and information would you give Helen?

(4) (a) Mr Laville is to have prostate surgery under general anaesthetic. His diabetes is usually well controlled on gliclazide 80 mg bd and metformin 500 mg bd. What care will Mr Laville require with regard to his diabetes?
(b) Mrs Parker has poorly controlled Type 2 diabetes. She usually takes gliclazide 160 mg, metformin 850 mg tds and acarbose 100 mg tds. She is due to undergo a coronary artery bypass graft in two months time. How should Mrs Parker's diabetes be managed?

For suggested answers see pages 255–6.

References

Ahmed AM (2000) Islamic pillars: possible adverse effects on diabetic patients. Practical Diabetes International, May 17(3): 96–7.

Alban Davies H, Clark JDA, Dalton KJ, Edwards OM (1989) Insulin requirements of diabetic women who breast feed. British Medical Journal 298: 1357–8.

Audit Commission (2000) Testing Times: A Review of Diabetes Services in England and Wales. London: Audit Commission Publication.

Balarajan R, Soni Raleigh V (1993) Ethnicity and Health – A Guide for the NHS. London: Department of Health/HMSO.

British Diabetic Association (BDA) (1992a) Driving and Diabetes. London: BDA.

British Diabetic Association (BDA) (1992b) Dietary recommendations for people with diabetes: an update for the 1990s. Diabetic Medicine 9(2): 189–202.

British Diabetic Association (BDA) (1997) Diabetes Care Today: A Guide for Residential and Nursing Home Managers and Staff. London: BDA.

British Diabetic Association (BDA) (1999) Guidelines of Practice for Residents with Diabetes in Care Homes. A British Diabetic Association Report. London: BDA.

Brown V (1997) Diabetic pregnancy: an inner city perspective. Journal of Diabetes Nursing 1(2): 45–9.

Brown CJ, Dawson A, Dodds R et al. (1996) Report of the Pregnancy and Neonatal Care Group Diabetic Medicine 13: S43–S53.

Burden AC (1996) Quality of care, past, present and future. Indo-Asian diabetes practical methods of improving care. Practical Diabetes International Supplement 13(3): S2–S3.

Burden AC, Samanta A, Rahman F (1991) Lessons from the Indian diabetic. Practical Diabetes 8(6): 224–6.

Chief Medical Officer (1992) On the State of Public Health 1991. London: HMSO.

Chief Medical Officer (1994) The Report on the Confidential Enquiries into Maternal Deaths 1988–1990. London: HMSO.

Clinical Standards Advisory Group (1994) Standards of Clinical Care for People with Diabetes. London: HMSO.

Connell CM (1991) Psychosocial aspects of diabetes and older adulthood: reciprocal effects. Diabetes Education 17: 364–71.

Coscelli C, Calabrese G, Fredele D, Pisu E, Calderini C, Bistoni S et al. (1992) Use of pre-mixed insulin among the elderly. Diabetes Care 15: 1628–30.

Coulston AM, Mandelbaum D, Reaven GM (1990) Dietary management of nursing home residents with non-insulin dependent diabetes mellitus. American Journal of Clinical Nutrition 51: 67–71.

Cousins L (1987) Pregnancy complications among diabetic women: review 1965–1985. Obstetrics and Gynecology 42: 140–9.

Cruickshank JK, Alleyne SA (1987) Black West Indian and matched white diabetics in Britain compared with diabetics in Jamaica. BM, BP and vascular disease. Diabetes Care 10(2): 170–9.

Davison JM, Lindheimer MD (1993) Renal disorders. In Creasy RK, Resnick R (Eds) Maternal Foetal Medicine: Principles and Practice. 3rd edn. London: WB Saunders, pp 844–64.

Department of Health (2001a) National Service Framework for Older People. London: The Stationery Office.

Department of Health (2001b) Care Homes for Older People. National Minimum Standards. Care Standards Act 2000. London: The Stationery Office.

Department of Health (2001c) National Service Framework for Diabetes Standards. London: HMSO.

Diabetes UK (2000) Recommendations for the Management of Pregnant Women with Diabetes (Including Gestational Diabetes). London: Diabetes UK.

Dornhorst A, Paterson CM, Nicholls JSD et al. (1992) High prevalence of gestational diabetes in women from ethnic minority groups. Diabetic Medicine 9: 820–5.

Douek I, Bowman C, Croxson S (2001) A survey of diabetes management in nursing care homes: the need for whole systems of care. Practical Diabetes International June 18(5): 152–4.

Dunlop DC, Kelly LC, Dunster GD, O'Hare JP (1997) Insulin dependent diabetic pregnancy and driving: is the correct advice being given? A telephone survey. Practical Diabetes International 14 (1): 12–13.

Elliot K, Fuller J (1991) Health education and ethnic minorities. British Medical Journal 302: 802–3.

Fox C, Pickering A (1995) Diabetes in the Real World. London: Class Publishing, pp 91–110.

Frost G, Annan M, Bebele J et al. (1992) Providing dietary advice for Afro-Caribbeans with diabetes. Practical Diabetes 9(3): 118–19.

Funnell MM (1990) Role of diabetes educator for older patients. Diabetes Care 13 (suppl. 2): 60–5.

Garner PR, D'Alton ME, Dudley DK et al. (1990) Pre-eclampsia in diabetic pregnancies. American Journal of Obstetrics and Gynecology 163: 505–8.

Gill GV (1997) Surgery in patients with diabetes mellitus. In Pickup J, Williams G (Eds) Textbook of Diabetes. 2nd edn. Oxford: Blackwell Science.

Girling JC, Dornhorst A (1997) Pregnancy and diabetes mellitus. In Pickup J, Williams G (Eds) Textbook of Diabetes. 2nd edn. Oxford. Blackwell Science, pp 72.1–72.34.

Goodwin AM, Keen H, Mather HM (1987) Ethnic minorities in British diabetic clinics. Diabetic Medicine 4: 266–9.

Govindji A (1991) Dietary advice for the Asian diabetic. Practical Diabetes 8(5): 202–3.

Govindji A (1992) A taste of the Caribbean. Balance February/March (BDA).

Govindji A (1996) Aims and goals of dietary advice. Indo-Asian diabetes: practical methods of improving care. Practical Diabetes International Supplement 13(3): S4–S5.

Griffith DNW, Yudkin JS (1989) Brittle diabetes in the elderly. Diabetic Medicine 6: 440–3.

Harris MI, Klein R, Welborne TA, Knuiman MW (1992) Onset of NIDDM occurs at least 4–7 years before clinical diagnosis. Diabetes Care 15: 815–19.

Hawthorne K (1990) Asian diabetics attending a British diabetic clinic – a pilot study to evaluate their care. British Journal of General Practice June: 243–7.

Health Education Authority (1994). Black and Minority Groups in England. London: HEA, Chapter 2.

Henry OA, Beisher NA (1991) Long term implication of gestational diabetes for the mother. Baillière's Clinical Obstetrics and Gynaeology 5: 461–83.

Hughes TAT, Borsey DQ (1994) The management of diabetic patients undergoing surgery. Practical Diabetes 11(1).

Husband DJ, Thai AC, Alberti KGMM (1986) Management of diabetes during surgery with glucose–insulin–potassium infusion. Diabetic Medicine 3: 69–74.

Jerreat L, Parker FC (1997). Protocols for the management of diabetics undergoing investigation. Internal document, Greenwich Healthcare Trust (unpublished).

Jones G (1996) Education about diabetes mellitus for Indo-Asians. Indo-Asian diabetes: practical methods of improving care. Practical Diabetes International 13(3, suppl.): S10–S11.

Kilvert JA, Nicholson HO, Wright AO (1993) Ketoacidosis in diabetic pregnancy. Diabetic Medicine 10: 278–81.

Kitzmiller JL, Gavin LA, Gin GD et al. (1991) Preconception care of diabetes: glycaemic control prevents congenital anomalies. Journal of the American Medical Association 265: 731–6.

Leslie D (1991) Genetic counselling in diabetes. In Pickup J, Williams G (Eds) Textbook of Diabetes. 1st edn. Oxford: Blackwell Science, pp 861–4.

McAvoy BR, Raza R (1991) Can health education increase uptake of cervical smear testing among Asian women? British Medical Journal 302: 833–6.

Marks L (1996) Counting the Cost: The Real Impact of Non Insulin Dependent Diabetes. London: Kings Fund Policy Institute/BDA.

Marsden P (1997) Protocol for the management of diabetes and pregnancy. Greenwich District Hospital (unpublished).

Mather HM (1991) Diabetes mellitus in ethnic communities in the UK. In Pickup J, Williams G (Eds) Textbook of Diabetes. 1st edn. Oxford: Blackwell Science, pp 909–11.

Meneilly GS, Tessier D (1995) Diabetes in the elderly. Diabetic Medicine 12: 949–60.

Meneilly GS, Cheung E, Tessier D, Yakura C, Tuokko H (1993) The effect of improved glycemic control on cognitive functions in the elderly patient with diabetes. Journal of Gerontology 48: M117– M121.

Odugheson O, Rone B, Fletcher J et al. (1989) Diabetes in the West Indian community: the Wolverhampton survey. Diabetic Medicine 6: 48–52.

Page RCL, Kirk BA, Fay T et al. (1996) Is macrosomia associated with poor glycaemic control in diabetic pregnancy? Diabetic Medicine 13: 170–4.

Palinkas LA, Barrett-Conner E, Wingard DL (1991) Type 2 diabetes and depressive symptoms in older adults: a population based study. Diabetic Medicine 8: 532–9.

Petterson T, Dornan TL, Albert T, Lee P (1994) Are information leaflets given to elderly people with diabetes easy to read? Diabetic Medicine 11: 111–13.

Royal College of Radiologists (1998) Advice to Members and Fellows with regard to Metformin induced Lactic Acidosis and X-ray Contrast Medium Agents. London: Royal College of Radiologists.

Samanta A, Burden AC, Jagger E (1991) A comparison of the clinical features and vascular complications of diabetes between migrant Asians and Caucasians in Leicester, UK. Diabetes Research in Clinical Practice 14: 205–14.

Schwartz R, Gruppuso PA, Petzolol K et al. (1994) Hyperinsulinaemia and macrosomia in the foetus of the diabetic mother. Diabetes Care 17: 640–8.

Shaukat N (1996) Coronary heart disease. Indo-Asian diabetes: practical methods of improving care. Practical Diabetes International 13(3, suppl.): S9–S10.

Sinclair AJ (1994) Diabetes care in the aged: time for reappraisal. Practical Diabetes 11(2): 60–3.

Sinclair A (1995) Initial management of non insulin dependent diabetes mellitus in the elderly. In Finucane P, Sinclair AJ (Eds) Diabetes in Old Age. Chichester: Wiley, pp 181–201.

Sinclair AJ, Barnett AH (1993) Special needs of elderly diabetic patients. British Medical Journal 306: 1142–3.

Steel J (1988-89) Hypos when you are pregnant. Balance December/January (BDA).

Steel JM (1994) Personal experience of pregnancy care in women with insulin dependent diabetes. Australian and New Zealand Journal of Obstetrics and Gynaecology 34: 135–9.

Stout RW (1997) Old age and diabetes mellitus. In Pickup J, Williams G (Eds) Textbook of Diabetes. 2nd edn. Oxford: Blackwell Science, pp 74.1–74.11.

Thompson DM, Dansereau J, Creed M et al. (1994) Tight glucose control results in normal perinatal outcome in 150 patients with gestational diabetes. Obstetrics and Gynaecology 83: 362–6.

Thomson FJ, Masson EA, Learning JT, Boulton AJ (1991) Lack of knowledge of symptoms of hypoglycaemia by elderly diabetic patients. Age and Aging 20: 404–6.

Tong P, Baillie SP, Roberts SH (1994) Diabetes care in the frail elderly. Practical Diabetes 11(4): 163–4.

Tun PA, Nathan DM, Perlmuter IC (1990) Cognitive and affective disorders in elderly patients with diabetes. Clinics in Geriatric Medicine 6: 731–46.

Watkinson M (2001) Should there be DSNs specifically for older people? Journal of Diabetes Nursing (4).

Weedon L, Curry M (1994) Diabetes monitoring for all? Practical Diabetes 11(1): 24–6.

Whichelow MJ, Dodderidge MC (1983) Lactation in diabetic women. British Medical Journal 287: 649–50.

Wilson E, Wardle P, Chandel P, Walford S (1993) Diabetes education: an Asian perspective. Diabetic Medicine 10: 177–80.

Ylinen K, Aula P, Stenman UH et al. (1984) Risk of minor and major foetal malformations in diabetics with high HbA1$_c$ values in early pregnancy. British Medical Journal 289: 345–6.

SECTION THREE
DIABETES CARE IN CONTEXT

Chapter 7
Psychological care

Diabetes has major psychological, social and physical implications for people's lives. The disease cannot be separated from the person with the disease. Psychological care is a vital part of diabetes management and should be an integral part of all consultations with health professionals. It should not just be reserved for those with 'problems' or for those who fail to 'comply' with treatment regimes. Although I have attempted to demonstrate the importance of psychological care throughout the book, I believe that it is so vital that it demands a separate chapter.

In this chapter I shall explore the psychological difficulties of living with diabetes. The effects of diagnosis, the relationship between those with diabetes and health professionals and counselling skills will be discussed. The problems of needle phobias and life crises will also be addressed. I have chosen to refer to the person with diabetes as both the patient and the client in this chapter. Despite the problems associated with the use of 'patient', I have used this term except when quoting or paraphrasing other authors or describing counselling situations when terminology from the social sciences seemed more appropriate.

Learning Outcomes

After reading this chapter you should be able to:

(1) demonstrate sensitivity to the psychological implications of diabetes;
(2) provide diabetes care which supports patient empowerment;
(3) recognize and set goals to manage psychological difficulties which may affect diabetes management.

The Psychological Implications of Diabetes

Diabetes is an incurable, lifelong condition. The demands of diabetes change and people need to adapt to these continually. For example, 'normal' life events such as pregnancy, holidays, intercurrent illness and bereavement may have dramatic effects on glycaemic control. Changes specific to the disease such as long-term complications or hypoglycaemic unawareness have major psychological implications.

Diabetes is invisible; a 17-year-old expressed a desire for people to see diabetes 'like a broken leg'. She felt that this might lead to greater understanding. She had been judged as being drunk by passers-by when hypoglycaemic after a party. Shillitoe (1994) suggests that diabetes has no external evidence that would excite sympathy, or any of the privileges or concessions usually extended to the sick. Diabetes may not even cause symptoms to some with Type 2 diabetes making diagnosis even more difficult to accept.

The management of diabetes is hard work for those with diabetes and requires behavioural change. These changes include changes in eating patterns such as having to eat when not hungry and at inconvenient times. Career changes may also be necessary (see p. 123) and there may be restrictions on driving. Planning becomes necessary for activities usually taken for granted, such as exercise, alcohol, meals out and shift work.

The skilled measurement of blood (or urine) glucose concentrations is necessary and knowledge is required to act on the results. Insulin injections may be necessary and venous blood samples will be necessary for screening purposes. These will be particularly difficult for those with needle phobias. Some people with diabetes may be unable or unwilling to make all these changes. According to Sarafino (1994) compliance with medical recommendations tends to be low when the regimen is complex, needs to be followed for a long period of time, requires changes to lifestyle or is designed to prevent rather than cure illness. The treatment of diabetes has all these characteristics.

Those treated with insulin or sulphonylureas live with the threat of hypoglycaemia. Unfortunately, the better controlled the diabetes is, the greater the risk of hypos. Many patients fear hypos. At the very least they can cause embarrassment and loss of control and hypoglycaemia may even lead to coma and death. Insulin and sulphonylureas may also lead to weight gain, another cause of distress to many.

There is also the shadow of diabetic complications. Although good control is associated with a reduction in risk (DCCT, 1993), there are no guarantees that good control will always prevent complications. Consider, for instance, those with Type 2 diabetes who may have had diabetes years before it was diagnosed, or the adult with Type 1 diabetes who lives with the fear that their adolescent years with poor diabetes control may yet affect them.

Stuart Bootle (1997) a GP, describes in *Balance* (the journal of the British Diabetic Association), how he had to weigh the fears for the future (complications) against the quality of life now. He had controlled his diabetes very tightly and had experienced recurrent hypos which had started to ruin his relationship with his girlfriend. Preventing the hypos meant that he had to face his fears of complications.

Self-confidence, a supportive family or friends and people prepared to help are cited by Shillitoe (1994) as necessary to achieve the flexibility required in managing diabetes. Kelleher (1988) cites Fletcher (1982), who attributed his successful management of diabetes for 40 years to the support received from his wife, in particular her ability to recognize a hypo:

> Once I clutched my wife saying 'The world is coming to an end and I want to hold on to you'. 'All right', she said 'but drink some Lucozade first'; and the world was saved. (p. 79)

Not everyone has a supportive family; diabetes itself puts enormous strain on family members, and many people with diabetes lack confidence in themselves and their ability to cope.

A person's self-confidence is not enhanced by health professionals who compare their achievements negatively with others in the clinic. One woman recounted such a conversation:

> I'm sure you can manage at least one blood test a day; I realize that the baby takes up a lot of your time but another lady in the clinic has a baby and five other children and she manages.

Articles in *Balance* that feature people who successfully and apparently effortlessly combine successful careers with good diabetes control do not always encourage those who are struggling to combine diabetes with the rigours of 'everyday life'.

There may be a fear of passing on diabetes to children and guilt if a child is actually diagnosed as having diabetes. Kelleher (1988) cites a young woman with Type 1 diabetes who was told that her 18-month-old daughter had diabetes:

> 'I come home and said to him [husband] "They reckon she's got diabetes". I just couldn't look at him when I said it because I thought he's going to say to me , "You're the one that's got it – you gave it to her", you know. And I was so scared of what he'd say.' (p. 24)

Whole-person Care

The person with diabetes and the diabetes itself cannot be separated. Both physical and psychological care are therefore necessary.

The Diagnosis

Individual responses to the diagnosis of diabetes will differ. I have encountered people who were relieved that it was 'only diabetes' and not cancer, and many who were relieved that at least there was a reason why they had been feeling so unwell. For others the diagnosis of diabetes may be devastating because of the thought of injections for life or negative experiences of family members with complications. Some may deny the diagnosis and still others may become depressed.

Box 7.1: Objectives of whole-person care (Shillitoe, 1994)

- to concentrate on the person not the disease
- to create a relationship in which patients feel safe and therefore able to explore their thoughts, feelings and behaviours
- to identify psychological issues which may influence how the patient reacts to diabetes and copes with treatment
- to help patients find ways of coping effectively with diabetes
- to increase patients' feelings of competence and confidence in their ability to manage diabetes
- to give patients a set of skills to help them manage their diabetes
- to help patients evaluate their management skills and to make changes where necessary
- to reduce patients' feelings of uncertainty and vulnerability concerning the future
- to help patients achieve as much independence as possible from health services
- to apply these aims to the family or other carers when relevant
(p. 7)

Coping strategies

The following coping strategies are common when trying to come to terms with diabetes. The presence of these behaviours may indicate that the individual has not yet accepted his or her diagnosis.

(1) Denial

Denial is a normal response to loss and is commonly used as a way of coping. An element of denial may be a healthy response. Unfortunately, for some, this may be extreme and may prevent behavioural change such as diet or monitoring.

(2) Obsessional behaviour

Some may feel very anxious about the diagnosis and the risk of diabetic complications and feel the need to be 'in control'. Frequent blood tests and insulin/tablet adjustments are made; every item of food, exercise and stress may be documented. Diabetes becomes the focal point of their lives and periods of poor diabetes control are often perceived as personal failure rather than as the nature of the disease.

(3) Projection

The responsibility of diabetes management may be projected on to friends, relatives or health professionals. For example, 'I have to cook my husband chips five nights a week. It's his fault that I can't lose weight, my sugars are high and that I will die of heart disease.'

The grieving process

The diagnosis of diabetes is often seen as the beginning of a grieving process. Coles (1996) claims that in the case of diabetes, people need to adjust to the loss of health, of independence and of freedom. He argues that diabetes can mean the loss of prestige, self-image and confidence. Perhaps the most well-known model of grieving is described by Kübler-Ross (1970). This is a linear model: the stages begin with denial and isolation and progress through anger and bargaining and finally to acceptance. This model is most usually applied to loss through death, although it is widely accepted as having a place in chronic illness. Kübler-Ross's model can help people to understand what they are experiencing, but it should not be seen as prescriptive. People's experiences may be quite different; we should therefore not impose these stages on them.

Tinlin (1996) contrasts grief after bereavement which causes a final disruption to a relationship with ongoing chronic grief or sorrow such as in the case of the birth of a disabled child. The presence of the disabled child serves as a constant reminder of the loss suffered. People with diabetes face constant reminders of their loss (blood tests, injections, etc.). They have a significantly changed lifestyle (restrictions on food/activities) and an uncertain future (complications).

Teel (1991) claims that chronic sorrow is a normal result of ongoing loss, and defines chronic sorrow as 'a recurring sadness interwoven with periods of neutrality, satisfaction and happiness'. Tinlin (1996) claims that health professionals are generally very good at understanding the acute phases of grief but may play down grief after years of diagnosis or assume that it is pathological. Nurses need to be empathetic and recognize the normalcy of chronic sorrow, enabling the person with diabetes to employ effective coping strategies. She argues that the experience of having diabetes may then change from one of perceived loss to one of personal growth.

Why me?

A common question asked at diagnosis is 'Why me?' Many feel that they must have done something to deserve diabetes. Common explanations include eating too much sugar, a punishment from God for a past sin, or 'a shock' such as a car accident. If patients believe they are being punished or have done something to deserve diabetes it will have consequences for their self-confidence and their perceived ability to cope with diabetes.

Personal meaning

Shillitoe (1994) claims that each patient has to find his or her own meaning for diabetes in order to make life understandable and predictable. What is important to one person may or may not be so to another. Values and priorities change in response to changing situations. Avoiding hypos at all costs when at school may change to achieving tight glycaemic control despite the increased risk of hypoglycaemia when pregnant.

The meaning given by individuals to diabetes is determined by their family background, cultural and social background, and existing knowledge of diabetes. Patients from different cultural or social backgrounds may view health in different ways (see p. 164). Existing knowledge may be positive, such as knowing about a professional sports person who has diabetes, or negative, for example a relative who died at a young age or fund-raising posters which emphasize complications.

Management of Diabetes

Two terms that are often used in health care are empowerment and compliance. Most books and journals claim that the patient should be encouraged to take responsibility for his or her diabetes and to participate actively in decision-making. As health professionals we may, however, find it difficult when people fail to 'comply' with our carefully designed treatment plans. Many referral letters to the department in which I work describe those with poor diabetic control as 'non-compliant'. This assumption is often made without attempting to find out why the treatment plan was not followed. Did a clear plan exist? Was the person with diabetes aware of it? Were goals negotiated? Was it achievable in the real world – did it take into account the patient's abilities, skills, understanding, financial/social situation and his or her health care beliefs? Perhaps the patient did 'comply' and the treatment did not work. The statement 'If it works the professional takes the credit and if it fails the patient is to blame' is often too close to the truth.

Compliance

Compliance implies the submissive patient doing what he or she is told by the health professional and fits in with the traditional medical model. This model sees the professional as the expert who identifies and solves problems and delivers care. Physical status barriers may reinforce the authority of the professional and the passivity of the patient. These include the professional sitting behind a desk and having a larger chair, the wearing of a uniform, the professional drinking coffee (without the patient doing so), the use of jargon and the use of judgemental language such as 'cheating'.

Lack of compliance with the professional's recommendations is seen as failure on the part of the patient. There is a belief inherent in this model that professionals can motivate change in the person with diabetes, who is less knowledgeable and therefore less powerful than the professional. There is also a lack of trust in a relationship in which the professional looks for evidence of 'cheating'.

There is evidence suggesting that the use of the medical model is ineffective, and the health professional's advice is often not taken (Simons, 1992). Hernandez (1995) found that the compliance approach was ineffective in promoting good learning outcomes for people with diabetes. Shillitoe (1994) claims that using the medical model is likely to result in a dissatisfied and poorly controlled patient who requires more frequent appointments. Some professionals continue to make recommendations that are so far removed from the patient's own circumstances that they are impossible to follow.

Empowerment

This model acknowledges that patients have the right to make decisions about their lives. Only the individual can decide whether the benefits of a management plan outweigh its emotional, social, physical, psychological and financial costs (Shillitoe, 1994). Empowerment gives patients the necessary skills and knowledge to allow them to work in partnership with the professional and make informed decisions about their management.

Empowerment has been termed a patient-centred model (Funnell et al., 1991). Using this model, diabetes is seen as a psychological and social condition rather than as just a physical disease. The problems and learning needs are identified by the person living with diabetes rather than the professional. The individual has the prime responsibility for his or her own health and has the ability to make and act on decisions, although information and help may be required from professionals (Gibson, 1991). The professional is therefore seen as a resource rather than a care-giver and problem-solver and shares rather than takes responsibility for setting goals for diabetes management. The professional has expertise in medical aspects of the condition, but the patient is the expert on how he or she wishes to live life and on the constraints on him or her. The relationship is two sided, based on mutual respect and trust. The patient's decisions (even if different from those which the health professional might have made for him or her) are accepted and valued.

Skinner and Craddock (2000) define empowerment as involving at least five key features: acceptance, affect, autonomy, alliance and active participation. In a nutshell acceptance refers to the respect that the health professional must have for the person with diabetes. Affect refers to exploring the emotions which the patient associates with the problem. Autonomy refers to the responsibility of the individual with diabetes for the content of the consultation. Alliance refers to the partnership between professional and patient and active participation refers to both parties who should be active. Although the patient is making the decisions, the professional should be involved in active listening and active questioning, helping the patient to identify areas for change and barriers to change, and establishing a commitment to change. Strategies to help use the empowerment approach will be discussed later in the chapter. Skinner and Craddock (2000) do admit that although intervention studies have tested some elements of the empowerment model, there is no published empirical study that has tested empowerment in its entirety. Arguments for the effectiveness of the patient empowerment model are therefore based on philosophical rather than evidence-based grounds.

Health professionals cannot empower patients. They can, however, help people with diabetes develop and use resources which promote a sense of control and self-efficacy (Gibson, 1991). Self-efficacy is how much an individual believes that he or she can influence, control or take charge of his or her life (Bandura, 1977).

Person-centred counselling is a stream of humanistic psychology and is influenced by the affluent culture in which it was devised in the 1950s and 1960s (Woolfe et al., 1989). Rogers (1961) sees the object of person-centred counselling as helping the *client* 'to become what he or she is capable of becoming' or using Maslow's terms (1962) to achieve 'self-actualization'. Woolfe et al. (1989) claim that these terms had a hollow ring about them in the Britain of the 1980s (and perhaps the 21st century), in which the social divide between the haves and have-nots is very apparent. They argue that striving for self-actualization is easier for those who are well off, well housed and have rewarding and secure jobs. Perhaps this may also be true of becoming empowered in terms of diabetes management. For those who are unemployed, poor or homeless, other objectives may assume a higher priority.

Beattie (1991) argues that if the empowerment approach is used in isolation in patient care without legislative action for health, it allows the well-established relationship between socioeconomic status and health inequalities (Townsend et al., 1992) to be overlooked and perhaps even condoned.

Working with patients as equal partners threatens traditional power structures and in the short term takes more time, which is usually in short supply. Some health professionals argue that patients want the professional to take control and simply want to be told what to do. This is true in some cases. Others argue that some patients are unable to understand the complexities of diabetes management and that patients do not ask questions because they do not wish to know, rather than because they feel threatened, or are given no opportunity in which to do so.

Patient empowerment has benefits for patients, including a positive self-concept, increased personal satisfaction, a sense of control and improved quality of life (Shillitoe, 1994). It is therefore more important in terms of time and resources than continuing to devise goals and plans which are so far removed from the patient's lifestyle that he or she is unable to follow them.

Later in this chapter I shall examine strategies to support patient empowerment, and counselling skills which can be used in diabetes care. First, however, I shall examine the effects of health care beliefs and attitudes on the control and management of diabetes.

Health Care Beliefs

Bradley et al. (1984) argue that the degree to which normoglycaemia is attainable is dependent on patient belief, including the degree to which the patient believes that blood glucose is controllable and the regime is worthwhile. Becker and Maiman (Becker, 1974; Becker and Maiman, 1975) modified the Health Belief Model (HBM). The HBM identifies four important belief factors which determine whether or not an individual will follow treatment recommendations. These beliefs concern perceptions of (1) the severity of the disorder; (2) vulnerability to the disorder; (3) benefits of treatment; and (4) the barriers to treatment. The HBM also claims that behaviour is triggered by 'cues to action' which make health threats more personal and obvious to the individual. These may be internal, e.g. symptoms of diabetes, or external, such as reminders from health professionals, family members or the media.

Bradley et al. (1984) developed a specific health belief scale related to diabetes. The barriers-to-treatment scale included statements such as 'controlling my diabetes well imposes restrictions on my whole lifestyle' and 'it is just not possible to control my diabetes properly and live in a way that is acceptable to me'. The benefits scale included 'regular controlled exercise helps in the management of my diabetes' and 'insulin reactions (hypos) can be prevented if I plan ahead'. Later, Bradley et al. (1987) expressed dissatisfaction with the vulnerability and severity scales, suggesting that interpretation was difficult. For example, a low vulnerability score may indicate ignorance or denial of the risks of diabetic complications or that, whilst aware of the general risks, the patient feels personally less at risk because of his or her efforts to improve control. Bradley et al. (1987) also pointed to the importance of interpreting the scores on these scales in the light of patients' beliefs about the complications which they may or may not already have.

Jenny (1984) compared compliance and health beliefs with the effects of age and duration of disease and argued that the importance of various aspects of the disease and regime is likely to change with age. Older patients saw diabetes as more serious and the middle-aged reported most barriers. The nature of the barriers changed with age; the elderly were most concerned about the cost of the diet and younger patients with blood/urine testing.

Brownlee-Duffeck et al. (1987) also reported age differences in health beliefs; in addition they found that the higher the perceived susceptibility the worse the metabolic control. There must therefore be other reasons why appropriate action has not been taken to control diabetes in spite of perceived susceptibility. Janz and Becker (1984) acknowledge that other factors in addition to beliefs influence health-related behaviours, including demographic variables, knowledge, perceived control, self-efficacy and social support.

Kelleher (1988) cites a young woman who had weighed up the costs and benefits of medical advice and the severity of and vulnerability to the disorder:

> I mean, I know that when I get to 70 or 60 or even 50 I'll go blind. I know I will. Or my leg will play up you know. Because I abuse my diabetes. But as I said, at least them 50 or 70 years I'm going to live happy. I'm not going to sort of say, oh I can't go shopping now because I've got to have [something to eat]. I just couldn't cope. (p. 52)

Locus of Control

Another psychological framework which has been used to attempt to understand the behaviour of people with diabetes is locus of control. This is a measurement of the extent to which a person believes he or she has control over important outcomes, such as his or her health. The notion of locus of control dates back to Rotter (1966). He identified alternative ways that people perceive control. First, internal locus of control, where individuals believe that they can influence outcomes, and second, external locus of control, where individuals regard events as the result of forces independent of their control.

Bradley et al. (1984, 1990) developed diabetes locus of control scales for insulin-treated and tablet-treated people with diabetes. They used subscales developed by Wallston et al. (1978) which distinguish between the dimensions of perceived personal control over health, perceived professional/powerful others' control and the perceived importance of chance factors.

Bradley et al. (1990) argued that a greater sense of personal control was associated with improved clinical and psychological outcomes, where opportunities for personal control existed. It was predicted that those scoring high on both personal and medical control and low on chance would have the best health status or diabetes control.

However, internal locus of control may become problematical when it means that it is impossible for an individual to see any event as due to chance or luck. Consider the person with internal locus of control who has adhered well to treatment and yet still develops complications. The emotional impact may be exacerbated when there is a stronger sense of personal control.

There would also be a discrepancy if a person with internal control who felt responsible for his or her health did not possess the necessary skills to translate the responsibility into action. Wallston et al. (1978) argue that this may lead to negative emotional states or defensive behaviours such as denial.

Strategies to Support Patient Empowerment

These are described by Shillitoe (1994) as key helper behaviours and include genuineness, respect, empathy and reassurance. Rogers (1978) describes three core conditions of the person-centred approach: congruence or genuineness, unconditional positive regard, and acceptance and empathy. He argued that these are therapeutic in themselves when communicated to the individual using communication skills.

Genuineness

We should attempt to be ourselves. Shillitoe (1994) acknowledges the temptations we may feel to keep our 'professional distance', either to protect ourselves from vulnerability or painful emotions, or because of the fear of being asked difficult and awkward questions or because of our own self-importance. It is important to be consistent and honest.

Consistency is not just saying and believing the same things at each visit. Our thoughts and feelings need to be consistent with the words which we use. There should be no falseness in the relationship. It is also important to treat different patients consistently. It is often easier to have more understanding towards someone who is attractive, polite or similar to ourselves. It may be more difficult to provide helpful suggestions or spend time with someone who identifies the same problem as the first patient but who smells, makes racist or sexist comments and is rude! Shillitoe (1994) claims that we need to be alert to these feelings and recognize the difficulties that they may cause in the formation of an effective helping relationship.

Honesty is also vital. If we do not know the answer to a patient's question we need to admit it and find out, not try to bluff our way out. Promises which cannot be met should not be made and patient misconceptions need to be corrected without making them feel stupid or confused. In order to be genuine, tact should coexist with directness (Shillitoe, 1994).

Acceptance and respect

Rogers (1978) describes this as having unconditional positive regard for the humanity of the client. It is not dependent on his or her behaviour. This may be difficult if patients behave in a way which we find hard to understand or accept. We all have our own biases and prejudices and we need to admit these to ourselves so that we can ensure that our behaviour with a patient is not adversely affected.

Empathy

Having empathy involves trying to see the world through the eyes of the patient, being able to identify with his or her experiences and communicating this understanding back to the patient. Unlike sympathy and compassion, empathy focuses on the feelings of the patient rather than our own feelings. In order to be empathetic, objectivity and skilled listening are required, which means looking beyond what the patient actually says. The basic message can be restated to the patient or summarized in a tentative way to check that we have understood. This gives an opportunity for the patient to correct any misconceptions or confirm our understanding. Empathy may pave the way for challenging a patient's point of view, setting goals, formulating strategies and moving to action (Egan, 1990).

Reassurance

Reassurance aims to promote patients' confidence in the treatment and in themselves. Giving information and explanations can be reassuring by reducing uncertainty. Showing interest and respect for the patient, staying calm and displaying confidence and competence are also reassuring. Shillitoe (1994) claims that reassurance is a set of skills and behaviours rather than the use of vague well-meaning words. The use of reassuring phrases such as 'It will all be all right – you'll see' usually means that the professional is avoiding the issues which are concerning the patient and showing neither respect nor empathy.

Counselling

Counselling is not just relevant in times of crisis. Developmental counselling can be used to help people anticipate the problems that lie ahead and therefore to become more independent and live more fully. Counselling involves helping people to help themselves, not solving people's emotional problems and relieving their hurt. Egan (1990) describes the goal of counselling in terms of helpers' effectiveness in the following way:

> Helpers are effective to the degree that their clients, through client–helper interactions, are in a better position to manage their problem situations and/or develop the unused resources and opportunities of their lives more effectively. (p. 5)

Egan (1990), however, does acknowledge that clients may not as a result of counselling manage their problems and opportunities better. They can choose not to!

Difficult types of problems may require different approaches and there are various schools of thought. These include person-centred therapy, Gestalt therapy, behaviourial therapy and cognitive therapy. All require the use of counselling skills.

A framework used frequently in diabetes care is based on that described by Egan (1990). This borrows ideas, methods and techniques systematically from all theories, schools and approaches and integrates them into a theory and practice of helping.

Egan's model progresses through three major stages: (a) the present scenario which allows explanation and clarification of the problem; (b) the preferred scenario, to help clients develop goals and objectives; and (c) getting there, to help clients develop action strategies for accomplishing goals, getting from the current to the preferred scenario. Each of these stages has 'three smaller steps' which Egan (1990) agrees in practice are not always clear and linear. When using the model, flexibility is essential; it should not be applied too rigidly.

Counselling skills

The terms and categories used are based on a counselling course which I attended in 1991 organized by Fox (consultant physician) and written by Gillespie (psychologist).

First contact

The first meeting with the patient and the beginning of the conversation can have a big impact on the future relationship. Our behaviour expresses our role and that of the patient. Initial contact should not be too formal; the counsellor should gesture to the patient where he or she should sit and should say how much time is available. Open sentences are important; these should be clear and inviting.

Box 7.2: Sentences to avoid

'What are your problems/difficulties?'
'How can I be of help?' (This undermines self-responsibility of the client and collaboration and may reinforce the client's view that he or she has a problem or is not coping)

Minimize expressions such as:
'Let's have a chat about…'
'Shall we start our little talk?'

Try instead:
'You wanted to talk with me [or your doctor suggested that you talk with me]; perhaps you can tell me what you have been thinking about?'
'You made an appointment to come and talk; we have until [state time]. Would you like to tell me what you would like to talk about today?'

Attending behaviour

This is used to make listening specific and observable; there are three key aspects to attending behaviour:

(1) *Eye contact:* It is important to look at someone if you are talking to him or her or listening. The counsellor should look for breaks in eye contact; if the client breaks eye contact his or her thoughts may be elsewhere.
(2) *Attentive body language:* Approximately 85 per cent of our communication is non-verbal. In Western culture the basic attentive listening posture is a relaxed easy posture with the trunk leaning slightly forward.
(3) *Verbal following:* The counsellor does not need to introduce new topics; the client should be allowed to do this and the counsellor should follow where the patient goes. In order for the session to be patient led, counsellors should not look for a solution or talk too much!

An example of verbal following is:

Client: 'I'm feeling really stressed out. The test I've got next week is really hard. What will my parents say if I fail?'
Counsellor: 'You feel tense, what does the test involve? You seem to feel under pressure by your parents to pass and you are worried about failing.'

Open invitation to talk – asking questions

The initial task of the counsellor is to find out what the client feels is a problem. This involves open questions. Open questions provide room for the client to express him or herself and usually begin with How, What, Could you, Can you. Closed questions come from the frame of reference of the counsellor and give the impression that the counsellor is trying to verify or formulate his or her own hypothesis. They do not allow the client to express him or herself and usually emphasize factual content rather than feeling. Closed questions can usually be answered in a few words or with a yes or no answer, and should be reserved for when specific factual information is needed.

An open invitation to talk can be useful in different situations:

(1) To begin an interview. For example, 'What would you like to talk about today?'
(2) To help get the client to elaborate. For example, 'Could you tell me a bit more about that?'
(3) To elicit examples of specific behaviour. For example, 'What do you do when you feel fed up?'
(4) To focus attention on the client's feelings. For example, 'How does that make you feel?'

The use of 'why' can be threatening and demands of the client an explanation for thoughts or actions before his or her feelings can be fully explored. Care should be taken not to ask multiple questions, or questions which have more than one part. For example: 'Do you think that the difficulties you have performing regular blood tests are because you dislike needles, you can't operate the machine or because it reminds you that you have diabetes?'

Judgemental questions should also be avoided; for example, 'Do you feel guilty about eating so much chocolate?' These types of questions will make the patient clam up and give the expected 'Yes' answer.

Minimal encouragers

These are indicators to another person that you are 'with' him or her and may help to keep clients talking. Non-verbal minimal encouragers include appropriate head nods, eye contact and the absence of distracting movements. Verbal minimal encouragers are brief utterances such as 'Oh?' and/or the repetition of one or two key words: 'tell me more', 'umm-hmmm', 'uh-huh' or simple restatement of the exact same words of the client's last statement. Silence is also an important minimal encourager; it frees the client to think, feel and express. If silence is helpful the client will continue; if not, basic attending and open questions can be used.

Paraphrasing

Paraphrasing repeats back to the client, in the counsellor's own words, pieces of information which the client has given. Paraphrases can be helpful in several ways:

(a) conveying to the patient that you are with him or her;
(b) crystallizing clients' comments, making them more concise;

(c) checking the accuracy of the counsellor's perceptions;
(d) giving direction to the interview.

A paraphrase is a tentative translation of what was said rather than parrot-like repetition. There is a difference between minimal encouragers and paraphrasing. For example:

> Client: 'I don't know what to do. One moment my blood sugar is too high the next it is really low.'
> Counsellor: (minimal encourager): 'Really low.'
> Counsellor: (paraphrase): 'It sounds as if your diabetes is really unstable at the moment.'

Reflecting feelings

Reflecting feelings shows that the counsellor is trying to understand what the client is experiencing emotionally. This ideally results in the client noticing that his or her feelings are accepted, and receiving attention, thus stimulating further disclosure and awareness of those feelings. Reflecting feelings is particularly important when clients have mixed feelings which inhibit them from getting a clear picture. Clients may express feelings both verbally and non-verbally. When reflecting feelings, it is important that the counsellor has the right intensity of feeling, not stronger or weaker than expressed by the client:

> Client: 'I can't ever get away from it; I have to carry sugar, an ID card, inject twice a day, eat regularly and test my blood if I don't I'm ill and that's even worse.'
> Counsellor: 'You sound very angry and frustrated about the way that diabetes affects your life.'

Concreteness

In order to set goals and begin problem-solving the counsellor and the client need to have a concrete view of what the problem is. The counsellor can stimulate the client to be more concrete by:

(1) asking concrete open questions such as 'What happened exactly?';
(2) interrupting vague rambling stories with concrete paraphrase, reflections and clarifying questions. For example:
    Client: 'Everything has gone wrong. I've got no friends at college and I can't do the work. I'm fat, my blood sugar is high and I feel ill, but if I up my insulin I just get fatter.'
    Counsellor: 'It seems like a lot of things are difficult for you at the moment. [paraphrase]. Shall we talk about each of these things one by one? What shall we discuss first? [concrete question].'

Ending the interview

Winding up

The interview should not be ended abruptly. As the allotted time is drawing to an end perhaps use a phrase such as 'We have only five minutes left; perhaps we can look at what we have talked about and make arrangements to meet again'. Patients often reveal important facts or questions at the end. It is important to acknowledge that the comment has been heard but not to rush to tackle it if there is inadequate time available. An arrangement to tackle the issue at the next meeting should be made. New topics should not be introduced by the counsellor at the conclusion; this gives the client the impression that he or she is free to continue for a while longer.

Setting goals

Goals should be identified by the client during the sessions and agreed between the client and counsellor as part of the counselling process. They should be relevant, realistic and achievable based on the patient's lifestyle, abilities and resources. Success increases self-confidence and motivation. The goals should be time limited and both the counsellor and the client need to be aware of the timescale involved. Time frames should be short, i.e. day-to-day, not lifelong.

The setting of goals or developing a preferred scenario is the second stage of Egan's model. The preferred scenario is a picture of the problem situation as it would be if improvements were made, not an idealistic state of affairs (Egan, 1990). For example, if the problem situation is a weight gain of two stones since insulin treatment, the preferred scenario may be no further weight gain or realistic weight loss of one pound per week. If a preferred scenario is complex then it needs to be broken down into interrelated subgoals. The client then requires help to choose a set of strategies which best fit his or her resources.

Summarization

Summarization attempts to help the client to clarify and pull together his or her thinking. In order to use summarization, the counsellor attends to the client's verbal and non-verbal statements over a period of time, selects critical issues and behaviour and re-states them as accurately as possible. This helps the client to see the situation more clearly. Summarization should be stated tentatively so that any distortion can be corrected by the client. When summarization is accurate it can move the interview from exploration to action and problem-solving. Summarizations cover a longer period of time than paraphrases and reflections of feeling and involve a broad range of issues. It is particularly useful if there have been previous meetings; the counsellor recaps the subjects discussed and clarifies what has been achieved. Summarization is also useful at the end of the interview when agreement is needed about the continuation of the sessions and to remind the participants of any management goals set during the session.

A behaviour change protocol

Anderson et al. (1996) and Skinner (1999) identify a behaviour change protocol using the empowerment model

- *Involve the patient; ask the patient to identify the problem.* What part of diabetes is the most difficult or unsatisfying for you?
- *Identify successes and failures.* When didn't you binge after dinner?
- *Negotiate a specific goal.* (this must be a behaviour that is achievable, realistic and measurable). How would this situation have to change for you to feel better about it? Where would you like to be in (specify time, e.g. six months)?
- *Assess how important it is to the patient for the situation to improve.* Are you willing to take action to improve the situation for yourself?
- *Identify strategies.* What are some of the steps that you could take to bring you closer to where you want to be? Are there barriers you would want to overcome? Are there people who could help you?
- *Formulate a contract.* Is there one thing that you will do when you leave here? A written commitment should be made.
- *Track progress.* Write down and record behaviour.

Needle Phobias

Although most people are not keen to self-inject or perform blood tests, the majority of people with diabetes manage very well. This is particularly true if clear explanations, demonstration of the technique and support are provided (see p. 110). Some patients are, however, needle phobic and are terrified and panic at the thought of injections. Some have avoided the dentist, or tropical holidays which require vaccinations.

The management of needle phobia uses methods from the behavioural school of psychology (see Box 7.3).

Shillitoe (1988) argues that method 10, which includes the use of relaxation, modelling and systematic desensitization, in imagination and real-life practice is most effective to overcome needle phobias.

Although these methods have been listed separately, in practice more than one method is usually used in any treatment programme.

I now discuss a true life case of needle phobia; only the name has been changed!

Case-study 7.1

Kevin is 52 years old and has Type 2 diabetes which was diagnosed 12 years ago. He is happily married with five children and eight grandchildren. His diabetes control has been deteriorating for the last two years and Kevin is taking maximal oral hypoglycaemic therapy. He is losing weight, thirsty and tired and has background retinopathy and neuropathy. Insulin therapy has been suggested.

Box 7.3: Behavioural methods (based on Shillitoe, 1988)

(1) Specific assignments which set explicit treatment goals
(2) Promoting and cueing specific behaviours. For example; telephone prompts to improve appointment keeping and tablet taking
(3) Tailoring the regime to the particular needs of the patient. For example, the modification of dietary recommendations to fit into a particular family's eating routine
(4) Contracts which describe the role of patients and others which may specify a reward for attaining the goal
(5) Graduated implementation of new behaviours in easily managed steps
(6) Modelling and imitation to learn from the behaviours of others. For example; the demonstration of blood testing by a skilled nurse (modelling) followed immediately by the patient practising under skilled supervision (imitation)
(7) Monitoring behaviours and outcomes relevant to treatment. For example, an improvement in the accuracy of blood testing as a result of feedback about the technique
(8) Skills training to develop new behaviours
(9) Reinforcement of appropriate new behaviours. For example, rewards such as praise and encouragement
(10) Counter-conditioning to replace maladaptive behaviours with more appropriate behaviours

---

Kevin agrees that insulin is the right treatment but he is terrified of needles. He remembers being frightened of the dentist as a teenager and now feels extreme fear and panic at the prospect of insulin. He finds it difficult to share his fears with anyone, including his wife. His childhood may be relevant to his needle phobia. Kevin remembers that his father died a painful death after contracting an infection, possibly through an injection while under treatment at either the dentist or the hospital. Kevin was aged $7\frac{1}{2}$ years when his father died.

Stage number 5 was achieved by arranging for our patient helper to demonstrate an 'actual' injection on himself. The only adaptation to the hierarchy was stage 10. Initially stage 10 was Kevin injecting another but as we worked through the points Kevin felt that the need for him to inject another was unlikely to occur, but that performing an injection whilst away on business or at a restaurant was likely to be necessary.

The length of time needed to work through the stages and the stages themselves vary from patient to patient. For example, some may feel more confident with regard to insulin injections than blood testing. In Kevin's case the hierarchy was negotiated at the beginning of March and by the end of April he had successfully self-injected in a restaurant. In June of the same year he managed to travel to the West Indies. Other patients have taken longer: for one gentleman the process took almost a year; interestingly, the process was speeded up when diabetic symptoms became severe and he really needed insulin.

Box 7.4: The agreed plan of action

(1) A 10-stage hierarchy of desensitization was negotiated with Kevin, beginning at his least problematic situation involving needles and working up to the most problematic
(2) Kevin was asked to discuss with his wife:
   (i) the death of his father and its effects
   (ii) his difficulty in sharing his feelings
   (iii) the treatment hierarchy and stages
(3) Kevin was taught physical relaxation techniques, including slow deep breathing exercises and imagining a peaceful scene when anxious
(4) Kevin was encouraged to recognize what happens to him physically when he panics
(5) A timescale was agreed to work through the hierarchy

Box 7.5: Kevin's hierarchy

The aim is to work from 0–10 until you feel OK at 10. Do not move on to the next stage until you feel OK with the previous stage.

0 = OK
10 = Panic

(0)
(1) Wife performing blood test
(2) Performing blood test yourself
(3) Imagine being given an injection
(4) Imagine giving yourself an injection
(5) Watch someone having an injection
(6) Having venous blood taken
(7) Preparing insulin syringe for injection
(8) Being given an injection
(9) Self-injecting insulin
(10) Performing an injection in another situation

Life Crisis/Complications

Periods of stress, change and crisis are bound to occur during a lifetime of diabetes. Some events such as exams, leaving home, job changes, marriage and parenthood may be predictable and can be prepared for. Others, such as unexpected bereavement, the diagnosis of another disease and degenerative diabetic complications, may be unpredictable. During any major event or life crisis the person with diabetes may experience a period of disruption to glycaemic control and altered psychological adjustment to diabetes. The counselling skills described earlier in this chapter will be vital at these times.

Shillitoe (1994) suggests that there are two general factors which determine how well people cope with change: (1) the availability of social support (2) the patient's level of self-esteem.

Support

Support may be practical and emotional, often both. It can be given by family members and by health professionals. Patient helpers or 'buddy schemes' and support groups may also be available in some areas.

Self-esteem

This is how we feel about and see ourselves and how we would like to be. It may be based on how we have been valued by others, our performance at work or school, sports achievements and interpersonal relationships. Diabetes may affect self-esteem. A high self-esteem is likely to make patients feel that they are worth the time and effort required to improve and maintain their health (Miller, 1983).

Active listening will help determine how patients see themselves. Negative comments about their achievements or jokes about diabetes may indicate low self-esteem.

Treating patients with respect, valuing their opinions and the identification of their strengths rather than concentrating on their weaknesses will help to improve self-esteem. Patients can be encouraged to think more positively about themselves by using sentence-completion exercises or devising lists of positive attributes either verbally or on paper. Brown (1996) suggests that the patient writes down five words or phrases which best describe him or her as a person. The patient should be asked to cross out any negative statements and replace them with positive statements. Shillitoe (1994) suggests completing sentences such as:

'One thing I like about myself is...'
'One thing I do very well is...'
'A problem I handled very well is...'
'A compliment that has been paid to me recently is...'
(p. 92)

The professional can help by providing patients with evidence of success and praising achievements. Management goals should be achievable; this increases patient motivation and confidence. 'Failure' should be seen as failure of the therapy and not of the patient.

Predictable changes/crises

The professional can help to prepare the patient practically and psychologically for predictable changes. The patient can be asked to identify specific concerns. For example, going away to university may bring up issues such as telling new people that he or she has diabetes, living a long way from home, unpredictable meal times, alcohol, etc. Strategies for dealing with these issues can be developed; for example, changing to a basal bolus insulin regime may give more flexibility with meal times, so the contact number of the local diabetes nurse may be reassuring. Planning for these changes acknowledges that they are difficult and may prevent a major crisis in terms of diabetes control or academic achievements.

Unpredictable changes/crises

The development of diabetic complications or hypoglycaemic unawareness may require major psychological adjustment to changed circumstances. Grief responses such as anger and denial commonly experienced at diagnosis may re-emerge accompanied by bitterness and despair. Other situations may lead to uncertainty where the professional is unable to give 100 per cent assurance. For example, 'Will my baby be normal?'; 'I've got background retinopathy, will I go blind?'. Sometimes even positive results or answers can lead to psychological disruption. A 22-year-old man developed microalbuminuria and the beginnings of renal damage. He was told that this would mean the inevitable development of renal failure in the future. ACE inhibitors (new at this time as preventive treatment for renal disease) were prescribed which reversed the situation. The clinic team were elated but the patient was distressed. He had adjusted to the prospect of renal failure and its inevitability and found this new information difficult, not least because no assurance could be given regarding the future development of renal disease. More psychological adjustment was therefore necessary.

So What Can We Do?

(1) Establish the patient's concerns. Observe non-verbal and verbal communication, use open questions, minimal encouragers and reflection.
(2) Legitimize the patient's uncertainty. Demonstrate empathy and acknowledge his or her feelings as normal and understandable.
(3) Use concreteness to establish a concrete view of the problems experienced by the patient and begin to make plans to discuss each concern one by one.
(4) If there is no clear answer to the question/problem say so, acknowledge the difficulty the patient may experience in hearing this and move on to suggest how risks can be reduced. For example, 'We know that the outcome of pregnancy can be improved with good diabetes control. Shall we look at ways of improving your blood glucose?'
(5) If we do not know the answer because it is not our area of expertise, refer on to a specialist and offer to explore and discuss their worries.

Referral on

Referral on to a psychologist, a member of the mental health team or a professional counsellor is necessary if:

(1) The health professional is 'out of his or her depth'; the problem demands greater expertise and experience than the health professional possesses.
(2) The patient presents a problem which is similar to an unresolved problem of the health professional's and no other member of the diabetes team is available or able to provide the necessary care.
(3) The patient does not seem to be moving on. The sessions appear to be going nowhere.
(4) A pathological psychological problem is identified, e.g. depression, severe eating disorder, etc.

We are fortunate to work closely with a clinical psychologist with an interest in diabetes. She has provided help and advice on how to approach various situations and has encouraged us to refer on when necessary. She has also fed back on how she and the patient are progressing and on the strategies used. This has helped us to develop our skills in this area.

I have been unable to discuss all psychological problems experienced by people with diabetes. However, the provision of 'whole-person care', acknowledgement of the psychological implications of diabetes, the use of strategies to promote patient empowerment, the use of counselling skills, encouragement and praise are useful in all situations.

National Service Framework

The NSF standards relevant to this chapter are shown in Box 7.6.

Box 7.6: NSF Standards

Standard 3: Empowering people with diabetes

(3)   All children, young people and adults with diabetes will receive a service which encourages partnership in decision-making, supports them in managing their diabetes and helps them to adopt and maintain a healthy lifestyle. This will be reflected in an agreed and shared care plan in an appropriate format and language. Where appropriate, parents and carers should be fully engaged in this process.

Standard 4: Clinical care of adults with diabetes

(4)   All adults with diabetes will receive high-quality care throughout their lifetime, including support to optimize the control of their blood glucose, blood pressure and other risk factors for developing the complications of diabetes.

Questions

(1) List five psychological implications of diabetes.
(2) Describe how you can enable patients to become empowered.
(3) Jessica is 20 years old and has had diabetes for one year. Recently she has not been doing any blood tests and she failed to keep her last diabetic clinic appointment. As a health professional how would you approach this?

Suggested answers may be found on pages 256–8.

References

Anderson RM, Funnell MM, Arnold MS (1996) Using the empowerment approach to help patients change behaviour. In Anderson BJ, Rubin RR (Eds) Practical Psychology. Alexandria: American Diabetes Association, pp 163–72.

Bandura A. (1977) Self efficacy: towards a unifying theory of behaviour change. Psychological Review 84: 191–215.

Beattie A (1991) Knowledge and control in health promotion: a test case for social policy and social theory. In Gabe J, Calnon M, Bury M (Eds) The Sociology of the Service. London: Routledge, pp 162–202.

Becker MH (1974) The health belief model and personal health behaviour. Health Education Monographs 2: 324–473.

Becker MH, Maiman LA (1975) Sociobehavioural determinants of compliance with health and medical care recommendations. Medical Care 3: 594–8.

Bootle S (1997) In Winn D (1997) Me, myself and I. Balance Magazine November/December (BDA).

Bradley C, Brewin C, Gamsu D, Moses J (1984) Development of scales to measure perceived control of diabetes mellitus and diabetes related health beliefs. Diabetic Medicine 1: 213–18.

Bradley C, Gansu DS, Moses JL, Knight G, Boulton AMJ, Drury J, Ward JD (1987) The use of diabetes-specific perceived control and health belief measures to predict treatment choice and efficacy in a feasibility study of continuous subcutaneous insulin infusion pumps. Psychology and Health 1: 123–32.

Bradley C, Lewis KS, Jennings AM, Ward JD (1990) Scales to measure perceived control developed specifically for people with tablet-treated diabetes. Diabetic Medicine 7: 685–94.

Brown FJ (1996) . Psychological care. In McDowell JRS, Gordon D (Eds) Diabetes: Caring for Patients in the Community. London: Churchill Livingstone, Ch 3, pp 37–59.

Brownlee-Duffeck M, Peterson L, Simonds JF, Goldstein D, Kilo C, Hoette S (1987) The role of health beliefs in the regime adherence and metabolic control of adolescents and adults with diabetes mellitus. Diabetes Care 3: 139–44.

Coles C (1996) Psychology in diabetes care. Practical Diabetes International 13(2): 55–7.

Diabetes Control and Complication Trial Research Group (1993) The effect of intensive treatment of diabetes on the development and progression of long-term complications in insulin dependent diabetes mellitus. New England Journal of Medicine 329: 977–86.

Egan G (1990) The Skilled Helper: A Systematic Approach to Effective Helping. 4th edn. Pacific Grove CA: Brooks/Cole.

Fox C, Gillespie C (1991) Diabetes Counselling Course 17–20 October 1991 (unpublished).

Funnell MM, Anderson RM, Arnold MS et al. (1991) Empowerment: an idea whose time has come in diabetes education. Diabetes Educator 17: 37–41.

Gibson CH (1991) A concept analysis of empowerment. Journal of Advanced Nursing 16: 354–61.

Hernandez C (1995) The experience of living with insulin-dependent diabetes: lessons for the diabetes educator. The Diabetes Educator 21(1): 33–7.

Janz NK, Becker MH (1984) The Health Belief Model: a decade later. Health Education Quarterly 11: 1–47.

Jenny JL (1984) A comparison of four age groups' adaptation to diabetes. Canadian Journal of Public Health 75: 237–44.

Kelleher D (1988) Diabetes: The Experience of Illness Series. Suffolk: Richard Clay.

Kübler-Ross E (1970) Death and Dying. London: Macmillan.

Maslow AH (1962) Towards a Psychology of Being. Princeton, NJ: Van Nostrand.

Miller JF (1983) Enhancing self-esteem. In Miller JF (Eds) Coping With Chronic Disease. Philadelphia: FA Davis.

Rogers CR (1961) On Becoming a Person. London: Constable.

Rogers CR (1978) Carl Rogers on Personal Power. London: Constable Robinson.

Rotter JB (1966) Generalised expectancies for internal versus external control of re-inforcement. Psychological Monograms 80: 1–28.

Sarafino EP (1994). Health Psychology–Biopsychosocial Interactions. 2nd edn. New York/Chichester: Wiley.

Shillitoe RW (1988) Psychology and Diabetes: Psychosocial Factors in Management and Control. London: Chapman & Hall.

Shillitoe R (1994) Counselling People With Diabetes. Exeter: The British Psychological Society.

Simons M (1992) Interventions related to compliance. Nursing Clinics of North America 27(2): 477–84.

Skinner C (1999) Psychology and diabetes. Unpublished lecture notes from MSc course in diabetes 29 October. Chelsea and Westminster Hospitals, London.

Skinner TC, Craddock S (2000) Empowerment: what about the evidence? Practical Diabetes International May 17(3): 91–5.

Teel CS (1991) Chronic sorrow; analysis of the concept. Journal of Advanced Nursing 16(11): 1311–19.

Tinlin J (1996) A time to mourn? Practical Diabetes International 13(3): 86–7.

Townsend P, Davidson N, Whitehead M (1992) Inequalities in Health. The Black Report and the Health Divide. London: Penguin.

Wallston KA, Wallston BS, Devellis R (1978) Development of the multidimensional health locus of control scales. Health Education Monographs 6: 160–70.

Woolfe R, Dryden W, Charles-Edwards D (1989) The nature and range of counselling practice. In Dryden W, Charles-Edwards D, Woolfe R (Eds) Handbook of Counselling in Britain. Guildford and Kings Lynn: Biddles.

Chapter 8
Diabetes care in the community

Cathy Parker

This chapter describes the development of diabetes care in the community since 1989. The schedule of content requirements for diabetes chronic disease management programmes is used as a framework for presenting information (General Medical Services Committee (GMSC, 1993: 4). Links are made throughout the chapter to the National Service Framework (NSF) standards, that have particular relevance for primary health care and diabetes (DoH, 2001a). Some clinical information related to screening procedures is included, and a description of nursing roles. It concludes with a description of several diabetes care settings.

Learning Outcomes

By the end of this chapter you should be able to:

(1) give information to patients related to the availability of diabetes nursing care in the community;
(2) refer patients to appropriate health care professionals in the community;
(3) advise patients on what diabetes care they could receive from their general practice.

Scene Setting

This section focuses on the environment in which nurses are employed to care for people with diabetes in primary health care settings. In 1990 the NHS and Community Care Act changed the NHS into an internal market (Department of Health (DoH), 1990) with fundholding practices, multifunds and district health authorities purchasing local diabetes services.

The General Practice Contract introduced in 1990 encouraged practices to establish chronic disease management programmes in diabetes and acknowledged the potential for employing practice nurses to monitor patients with diabetes. A content requirement schedule for the Diabetes Mellitus Chronic Disease Management Programme included 10 items that influenced nursing activities within general practices (Box 8.1) (GMSC, 1993). These items continue to be highly relevant to the delivery of all diabetes services.

The NHS (Primary Care) Act 1997 introduced new contractual arrangements for the employment of GPs. Personal Medical Services (PMS) pilots were non-mandatory experiments, concentrated in inner city and other deprived areas. PMSs continue to multiply in number, but not all practices include diabetes care in their protocols (Lewis and Gillam, 1999).

Publication of *The New NHS – Modern, Dependable* (DoH, 1997) heralded the Labour government's reorganization of the NHS. The document signalled the end of GP fundholding and multifunds and the inception of a number of significant initiatives that have impacted on diabetes care (see Table 8.1).

Box 8.1: Content requirements of diabetes chronic disease management programmes

1   A register
2   Call and recall
3   Education for newly diagnosed people with diabetes
4   Continuing education for diabetics
5   Individual management plan (personal care plan)
6   Clinical procedures
7   Record keeping
8   Referral policies
9   Audit
10 Professional links

Table 8.1: Initiatives that have influenced diabetes care since 1997

1998	Health Improvement Plans
1998	Personal Medical Services
1999	Primary Care Groups established, subsuming GP fundholding Creation of National Institute for Clinical Excellence Creation of Commission for Health Improvement Total Purchasing Pilots
2001	Primary Healthcare Trusts established National Service Framework for Diabetes – standards document, published

Since the creation of Primary Care Groups in 1999 and latterly the progression to Primary Care Trust (PCT) status, primary care has been awarded decisive influence over the local diabetes services. Local Diabetes Services Advisory Groups (LDSAGs) exist in some, but not all areas. The creation of LDSAGs was inspired by Diabetes UK (formerly the British Diabetic Association) and represents a strategy for encouraging local stakeholders in diabetes care to interact in the planning and provision of high standard, comprehensive services based on local needs. LDSAG membership includes hospital specialist staff, primary care staff and patients. Overall, general practitioners have been providing an increasing proportion of diabetes care. Patients with complications or acute problems may be referred to specialist hospital services.

It is difficult to generalize about the features of diabetes services. The services have evolved over the last two decades, often along highly individual lines, dictated by local environs and resources. Hospital services are likely to comprise clinics in which doctors, dietitians, podiatrists and nurses provide a mixtre of clinical screening, monitoring and education. Diabetes Day Care Centres (DDCCs) tend to have a predominant role in the education of patients, urgent problems and 'day-to-day' management of individual patients. Diabetes Specialist Nurses are likely to be based in DDCCs.

The NSF for Diabetes provides service models for each of the 12 standards. This standards documents has subsumed the items from the diabetes chronic disease management programme and it emphasizes the need for equity of provision to include the monitoring and maintenance of minimum standards of care (see Appendix 3) (DoH, 2001b).

Standard 1 (DoH, 2001a) has particular implications for primary case based initiatives. It specifics that: 'The NHS will develop, implement and monitor strategies to reduce the risk of developing Type 2 diabetes in the population as a whole and to reduce the inequalities in the risk of developing Type 2 diabetes'. At the time of writing the implementation recommendations for the NSF have not been published, but initiatives along very similar lines to those already in place for the CHD National Service Framework are appropriate (Box 8.2).

Box 8.2

- HimPs (health improvement programmes) to be vehicles to develop partnerships between public health, health promotion personnel
- Local Equity Profiles to identify location of high risk populations: ethnic groups with high incidence of diabetes, etc.
- Health Impact Assessments

General practices can identify those most at risk of developing diabetes from parameters such as ethnicity, family history of diabetes, history of gestational diabetes, obesity and hypertension. Lifestyle advice, particularly on exercise, may help to delay or avert the onset. Dietetic advice aimed at reducing weight is another potential strategy.

Standard 4 of the NSF identifies the requirement to provide high quality clinical care for adults with diabetes (DoH, 2001a). The content requirements for the chronic disease management programme will now be used to structure the presentation of issues for diabetes nursing in primary case.

(1) Register

A practice diabetes register is the linchpin for the organization of a GP clinic. Registers should, ideally, be computer based. They can fulfil a number of functions if they are accurate and contain relevant data (Box 8.3).

Box 8.3: Functions of a practice diabetes register

- Recall system
- Check on the provision of comprehensive, equitable care
- Audit tool
- Record system

The NSF also contains a section on registers. In the short term a core data set is being developed and GPs will participate in the entry and codification of patient numbers and details on a practice or centre register. The NHS Information Authority is developing a nationally based specification, closely linked to coronary heart disease and stroke, which will structure the gathering of data and increase the scope for collation and comparison of data. The existence of a district wide register is an imperative. A register can be used for strategic planning of services and audit. The content of practice or centre registers is a crucial source of information for local health needs assessments that form a cornerstone for the implementation of the NSF. The software used to record data should, ideally, be compatible for use by all health care professionals working within the same district.

Box 8.4: Minimum data suggestions for recording on a practice register

A minimum data set entered on a practice register should contain information required to monitor NSF standards:

- Name, date of birth
- Duration of diabetes
- Treatment
- Complications
- Whether the patient is under sole or shared care

Source: Adapted from MacKinnon (2001: 69).

MacKinnon (2001) stated that a comprehensive register should contain details of what type of treatment the patient is receiving, risk factors, existing problems or complications and dates of most recent screening tests.

(2) Call and recall system

Easy, swift recall of data is the prerogative of computer-based systems with appropriately structured software. A call and recall system can be simple and effective. Manual systems for organizing the annual recall of patients are based on the patient's month of birth or on recalling all patients with surnames beginning with a group of alphabetical letters on specific months.

(3) Education of newly diagnosed people with diabetes

Coles (1989) described the need to create in patients the desire to know what they need to know. Topics covered by nurses in the community on the first appointment should be addressed according to what the patient needs to know in order to be safe. Subsequent topics should be addressed in an order prompted by the patient's questions and not because they are next on an educational check-list (see Chapter 4).

Coles also described the risks of 'pot-filling' style education, whereby health care professionals treat new patients as empty pots waiting to be filled with information. The information is dispensed in large quantities and too fast so that much of it is not retained. The patient's shock at being told that he or she has developed diabetes may act as a barrier to the retention of information. Counselling may be more appropriate at this stage. Comprehensive records should be kept of what topics have been discussed with patients.

(4) Continuing education of people with diabetes

The Diabetes UK leaflet *Diabetes Care – What You Should Expect* (British diabetic Association (BDA), 1997a) states that once reasonable control has been achieved, and when they are ready, patients should have more educational sessions. Standard 3 in the National Service Framework for diabetes (DoH, 2001a) states that structured education is a key intervention. This is to be individually tailored and utilize a skills-based approach. Nurses should assess existing knowledge of diabetes and explore patients' concerns or fears. The provision of a written record of all of the information given to the patient is essential.

The main areas to be covered by educational programmes are: nature of diabetes, the day-to-day management of diabetes, special problems and living with diabetes (BDA, 1997b).

(5) **Personal care plan (individual management plan)**

The Clinical Standards Advisory Group (CSAG, 1994) referred to individual management plans. The NSF (DoH, 2001a) changed the name and refers to' personal care plans as an aid to empower patients.

Diabetes UK (BDA, 1997b) referred to the need to identify individual targets for weight, blood glucose, blood lipids and blood pressure. These targets must be agreed with the patient. An 'ideal' target may not, in the patient's perspective, be achievable. The existence of an agreed plan is likely to involve the commitment of staff resources. Plans are officially endorsed as a strategy for use in the diabetes NSF.

(6) **Clinical procedures**

The main aim of many clinical procedures is to assess the patient with diabetes for existing or potential problems. Screening procedures are carried out in order to assess glycaemic control and risk factors that may render people with diabetes more liable to complications. Screening procedures also aim to detect complications at early stages.

Standard 4 of the NSF refers to the need to support the maximal control of blood glucose levels, blood pressure and other risk factors linked to the development of complications (DoH, 2001a). Standard 11 also requires the detection and management of long-term complications.

Screening

Diabetes Care – What You Should Expect outlined screening requisites on an initial and thereafter annual basis (BDA, 1997a). The role of nurses working in the community is likely to include some tasks relating to screening. The range and degree of involvement of nurses in screening procedures are subject to variations according to local policies, organizational structures, role specifications and individual expertise.

Clinical guidelines make specifications for the roles of nurses in screening procedures (Royal College of Nursing (RCN), 1994; BDA, 1997b). Under the terms of the chronic disease management programme each general practice submits a protocol to its Health Authority (until 1995 referred to as Family Health Service Associations). These protocols should have included details of nursing responsibilities. Integrated Care Pathways have in more recent years presented opportunities for local identification of 'who does what and when' (Hillingdon NHS Primary Care Trust, 2001).

Involvement of nurses in screening

Nurses undertake clinical procedures used to screen patients during initial assessments, annual and routine reviews (BDA, 1993).

Initial assessment following diagnosis

It is necessary to carry out a wide range of procedures in order to assess a new patient with diabetes. Bearing in mind that education and counselling will also be priorities for newly diagnosed patients, the initial screening procedures are likely to be spread out over several visits. Some of these initial procedures are also standard procedures for annual and routine reviews. The individual requirements of patients will decide the frequency of repeated procedures.

Diagnostic laboratory glucose estimations

Several authors have found evidence of spurious diagnoses of diabetes. Patchett and Roberts (1994) found that 10 patients attending their practice clinic had been given false positive diagnoses of diabetes. These patients may have had impaired glucose tolerance (IGT) at the time of diagnosis. The risk of spurious diagnosis also exists if based on inaccurate results produced by using blood glucose meters rather than laboratory blood glucose estimations.

It is difficult to confirm a diagnosis of diabetes from blood glucose estimations when patients restrict carbohydrate intake (possibly because of premature dietary advice from professionals) in the days prior to the test. Results may be within the normal or IGT range despite the existence of diabetes. Diagnostic guidelines must be strictly adhered to: if symptoms are not present, abnormal blood glucose results must be obtained on two different dates.

Review of risk factors

The NSF standard 2 requires GPs to employ strategies to identify people with diabetes who do not know that they have the condition. Factors associated with a higher risk of developing diabetes include a family history of diabetes, ethnicity (southern Indian, Afro-Caribbean), a history of gestational diabetes and obesity.

Any review of diabetes risk factors should include a calculation of coronary heart disease risk (British Hypertension Society, 2002). The coronary heart disease (CHD) guidelines for the CHD NSF include requirements for general practitioners in standards 3 and 4 (Box 8.5) (Department of Health, 2000).

Box 8.5: Standards applying to GPs for preventing coronary heart disease in high risk patients

General practitioners and primary care teams should:

Standard 3   Identify all people with established cardiovascular disease and offer them comprehensive advice and appropriate treatment to reduce their risks.

Standard 4   Identify all people at significant risk of cardiovascular disease but who have not developed symptoms and offer them appropriate advice and treatment to reduce their risks.

Reviews of risk factors in people with diabetes can identify indicators for inclusion in personal care plans.

Family history

History-taking should include finding out whether any close members of the patient's family have diabetes (and if so what type it is), cardiovascular disorders or hypertension.

Weight

All patients should be weighed. This provides an opportunity to discuss whether any weight loss has occurred over the last few weeks or months. If weight loss has been spontaneous and rapid, this gives an indication of whether the patient has Type 2 or Type 1 diabetes. Many nurses in the community are required to calculate the body mass index (BMI) of the patient in order to assess the degree of obesity (see Chapter 2, p. 23).

Blood pressure (BP) measurement

The increased prevalence of hypertension in people with diabetes is important because of its role in the development or acceleration of macrovascular and microvascular complications (Feher, 1993). Seventy per cent of patients presenting with Type 2 diabetes have a BP of more than 140/90 mmHg (Ramsay et al, 1999).

Two separate elevated readings are required to confirm a diagnosis of hypertension. Use of the 'alternative adult' cuff size (12.5–13.0 cm wide, 35 cm long) in all adults is recommended. Lower levels of intervention have been set for people with diabetes. Lifestyle advice may be beneficial, but it is now accepted that at levels of 140/90 for patients with Type 1 diabetes and 160/90 for patients with Type 2 diabetes, pharmacotherapy may be introduced (Keen, 1994). Target BPs for patients with proteinuria are lower than for those patients who do not have diabetes (Ramsay et al., 1999). Optimal first line therapy is not yet established for Type 2 diabetes, but trial evidence supports the use of ACE inhibitors, beta blockers, dihydropyridine, calcium channel blockers, alpha blockers and low dose thiazide diuretics (Ramsay et al., 1999). One-third of patients in the Hypertension Optimal Treatment study required three or more drugs in combination to achieve optimal control. The use of aspirin in all patients with diabetes and hypertension is also recommended (Ramsay et al., 1999).

Lipids

Diabetes is a risk factor for CHD. Random total and HDL cholesterol tests are carried out initially; repeat tests to confirm abnormalities are preferably from a fasting blood specimen. Triglycerides are also measured; raised levels are associated with poor glycaemic control and a higher risk of CHD (Garg, 1994). Target levels are < 5 mmol/L for total cholesterol, > 1.1 mmol/L for HDL cholesterol, < 3.2 mmol/L for LDL cholesterol and < 1.7 mmol/L for fasting triglycerides.

Smoking

A smoking habit within 5 years of carrying out a CHD risk assessment is a factor in the development of CHD (Department of Health, 2000). Practice nurses, nurse practitioners and health visitors are all likely to have experience of helping people to stop smoking as a part of their health promotion activities. All people with diabetes who smoke should be priority candidates for smoking cessation programmes.

Alcohol intake

Record alcohol intake in weekly consumption of units. Alcohol may be high on patients' educational agendas. Information should include reminders of prolonged hypoglycaemic effects when combined with sulphonylureas or insulin, and its high calorie content. The recommended top limit for daily intake is 3–4 units for men and 2–3 units for women.

Investigations

In addition to an assessment of risk factors, a number of initial tests and detailed individual assessments are necessary.

Ketonuria

The initial assessment at diagnosis has already been covered. It is worth repeating that it is crucial to exclude the risk of ketoacidosis by checking a urine specimen for ketones. The presence of moderate or large amounts of ketones would suggest that the patient may have Type 1 diabetes and hence the need for emergency referral to hospital.

Glycosuria

Concurrent checks on glycosuria and blood glucose level may indicate the presence of renal glycosuria or abnormal renal thresholds, rendering urine testing an unreliable method of self-monitoring. This applies particularly to the elderly.

Proteinuria

It is also necessary to check for the presence of protein in urine. Testing for minute amounts of protein in the urine (microproteinuria) has been advocated (Donnelly et al., 2000). Strip tests (Micral, Microalbustix) require samples of urine to be collected, preferably early in the morning. Results are obtained from a dipstick type test. Albumin/creatinine ratios performed by a laboratory and obtained from an overnight or timed collection of urine are a reliable and cost-effective alternative.

Blood tests

In addition to diagnostic glucose estimation, a venous blood specimen should be obtained and tested in order to establish other baseline measurements (Box 8.6).

Box 8.6: Suggested initial blood tests

Test	Reason	Further information
Glucose	Establish diagnosis	Laboratory specimen for diagnosis
HbA1$_c$, HbA1 or fructosamine	Monitor glycaemic control	At least annually
Urea & electrolytes, serum creatinine	Establish advisability of prescribing oral hypoglycaemic agents	At least annually
Liver function tests	Establish advisability of prescribing oral hypoglycaemic agents	Repeat as required according to medication. If not on medication and normal on first occasion repeat after a maximum of 5 years
Fasting lipids or total cholesterol	Indicator for increased risks of macrovascular disease	Every 3 years if normal
Thyroid function tests	Indicator for increased incidence in diabetes	Annually when antibodies present or problem exists
Full blood count	Detection of anaemia, haemoglobinopathy, infection	Abnormalities render HbA1$_c$ unreliable; infection causes raised blood glucose levels

---

Diet (see also Chapter 2)

Individual assessments are essential. Preliminary advice should include the need to reduce foods that are high in sugar and to spread out the carbohydrate intake.

Eyes

Visual acuity

Carry out a visual acuity test when convenient after diagnosis and annually thereafter. Use the initial result as a benchmark to measure any deterioration. An opportunistic test carried out by a nurse may be the only check obtained on patients who fail to attend for testing elsewhere. Housebound people with diabetes may also not otherwise be tested.

As regards equipment, 3 or 6 metre Snellen charts are used. Three-metre charts permit testing at a distance of 3 metres in smaller premises. Charts displaying non-alphabetical symbols are available for people who cannot read English alphabetical letters. Pictures need to be culturally appropriate for the person being tested.

How to do it

It is always necessary to record the patient's corrected vision, that is the size of letter that the patient can read when they are wearing their distance glasses (if needed). If the patient is unable to read the letters that have the number 9 underneath them (whether or not they are wearing distance glasses) then a pinhole device should be used (Taylor and Perkins, 1996). If the patient is unable to read even the largest letter then he or she should be moved half the distance towards the chart. This establishes the patient's vision at a distance equivalent to 3 metres from the chart. If the patient is unable to read the letter at the lesser distance, the tester should hold up the fingers of one hand (at a distance of 1 metre) and ask the patient to count the number of fingers. If unable to do this, the patient is asked whether he or she can see the tester making hand movements. If not, a pencil torch is shone into the affected eye, to check light perception.

Additional information about interpreting and recording the results is given in Box 8.7.

Box 8.7: Interpreting and recording visual acuity results

- Record the result as two numbers in fraction style; that is 6/18

- The top number recorded on the result indicates the distance from which the patient can read the letters; that is 6 or 3 metres

- The bottom number to be recorded is the number written in print underneath the smallest line of letters that the patient can read. This number indicates at what distance the person with normal vision would be able to read those letters

- Record ability to count fingers as CF (counts fingers), to see hand movements as HM, to perceive light as PL and unable to perceive light as NLP

Referral policy

Some practices have a policy of referring the patient to an optician if the vision has deteriorated by 'one line' over the period of a year (for example from 6/6 to 6/9). Immediate referral to an ophthalmologist may be the policy when a 'two-line' deterioration has occurred (for example from 6/6 to 6/12) (MacKinnon, 2001).

Ophthalmoscopy

The fundus comprises the retina, optic disc, macula and retinal vessels of the internal eye. The fundus is visible with an ophthalmoscope (Gilchrist et al., 1992). Ophthalmoscopy is necessary initially and then on an annual basis. GPs, nurse practitioners and optometrists (free test) perform the procedure.

Subsequent to examination, apply one drop of mydriatic solution (tropicamide 0.5 or 1 per cent) to the everted lower lid of each eye. The pupil dilates over about 20 minutes and the effect lasts for up to 6 hours. Patients should be warned prior to the appointment that they will be unable to drive for the rest of the day.

Foot care

Individual assessments are essential, at an appropriate stage following diagnosis. Day et al. (1987) made a distinction between the examination and inspection of feet. Foot examinations were a medical responsibility, whereas inspections were a nursing function.

Foot inspection

Foot inspections are carried out initially and at each visit by all practice nurses (RCN, 1994). An inspection consists of the general condition of feet including identification of sores or corns, etc., referral to podiatry as necessary and foot care education. Health care professionals should inspect feet that are prone to further complications at every visit. Patients should be asked to inspect their own feet daily (Skinner, 1996) (Box 8.8).

Box 8.8: Components of foot inspection

- Presence of structural deformities
- Colour
- Condition of the skin and nails
- Oedema
- Existence of callus and corns
- Footwear

Foot examination

The CSAG (1994) definition of foot examinations is: the assessment of foot deformities, peripheral foot pulses, vibration and sensation, foot ulceration and neuropathy. Foot examination is carried out as part of the formal annual review.

Nurse practitioners receive additional training in how to examine feet and check reflexes. An increasing number of district nurses and practice nurses are also learning how to palpate pedal pulses or use a doppler and to check for loss of sensation and vibration. These skills are used to assess housebound people with diabetes if GPs delegate the task of annual review to nurses.

Sensation

The availability of Semmes-Weinstein monofilaments has provided a valuable educational tool as well as screening equipment. A 10 g filament is sufficient for the purpose of identifying areas of lost sensation (Klenerman et al., 1996). The filament is used to identify the patchy nature of lost sensation and the patient advised to inspect these areas at least once a day (Figure 8.1).

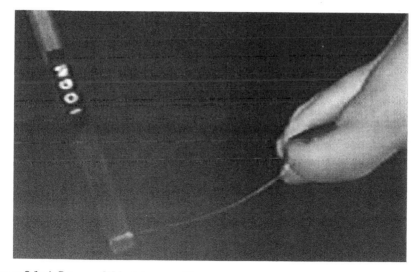

Figure 8.1: A Semmes-Weinstein monofilament

Press the filament against a selection of areas on the dorsal and plantar aspects of the foot. The filament bends when 10 g of pressure is applied. If there is no neuropathic damage the patient should be able to feel the filament.

Vibration

Use a 'C' tuning fork CO128. Check perception by placing the base of the vibrating fork on the tip of the big toe and ask the patient if he or she can feel the sensation. If the patient does not feel the vibration repeat further up the foot and leg, testing on the malleolus and the head of the tibia.

Fox and Pickering (1995) have offered tentative suggestions concerning qualitative foot problems and interventions by primary health care professionals (Table 8.2).

Table 8.2: Foot problems and interventions

Problem	Intervention
Loss of vibration sense; absent pulses without pain	Education
Callus or deformity	Podiatrist
Neuropathic ulcer	Podiatrist and diabetologist
Absent pulses, claudication	Vascular surgeon
Absent pulses, rest pain, discoloration	Urgent referral to vascular surgeon
Infected ulcer	Urgent admission
Pre-gangrene and gangrene	Urgent admission

Source: Adapted from Fox and Pickering (1995).

Annual Reviews

McDowell and Gordon (1996) described the 'annual review' as the 'MOT': a single annual visit when screening for complications is undertaken. Annual reviews should be offered to each person with diabetes. This review provides an opportunity to carry out checks on metabolic control and the patient's psychological, emotional and social well-being.

Many of the procedures outlined for initial assessment are repeated during an annual review (see Box 8.9).

Routine Reviews

A routine review should include all parameters that require review more frequently than on an annual basis. The reasons for routine reviews are likely to involve either review of personal targets, including the improvement of metabolic control, review of risk factors or complications identified at initial assessment, or annual review. The interval between reviews will depend on a number of factors (see Box 8.10).

At routine reviews comprehensive physical examinations are not carried out and investigations are requested as required.

> **Box 8.9: Annual review**
>
> - Initial discussion
>   Enquiries about: lifestyle, glycaemic control (inspection of patient's blood or urine testing results), existing understanding of diabetes and symptoms
>
> - Educational review
>   Further information relating to diabetes and self-care that the patient requests
>
> - Examination
>   Weight, blood pressure, eyes, feet, reflexes, injection sites (if applicable)
>
> - Investigations
>   Urinalysis, microalbuminuria or albumin/creatinine ratio
>   Blood test for HbA1$_c$ or fructosamine; serum creatinine, urea and electrolytes, fasting lipids (serum cholesterol 3-yearly if previous result normal), thyroid function (if applicable)
>
> - Individual management plan
>   Negotiation of targets with the patient for weight and BMI, glycaemic control, alcohol intake, smoking and exercise
>   Adjustment or changes to prescribed medication
>   Book next review appointment
>   Refer to dietitian, podiatry, ophthalmologist, specialist diabetes nurse, hospital diabetic clinic, male sexual dysfunction clinic, family planning or pre-pregnancy clinics, etc., as indicated
>
> *Source:* Adapted from BDA (1997b).

> **Box 8.10: Factors influencing frequency of reviews**
>
> Overall metabolic control   Change of therapy during previous visit
> Complication status   Educational requirements

Record keeping

All clinical results should be recorded on computer or on a diabetes record card (Figures 8.2–8.5). The NSF (DoH, 2001a) endorses the provision of patient-held records as a method for facilitating self-care. The existence of patient-held records may help to avoid unnecessary duplication of tests for patients whose care is shared between their general practice and a hospital diabetes clinic.

The NSF for Diabetes – Delivery strategy (DoH, 2003) has stressed that these records should include an agreed care plan, including education and personal goals for the person with diabetes. The record should also identify the person(s) responsible for the delivery of care.

DIABETIC REVIEW CARD

Name	D.O.B.
Address	NHS No
	Hosp.
Tel.	Hosp No.

Language spoken:

Language read:

DIABETIC HISTORY

Age at diagnosis   F.H.
Initial presentation and treatment

Initial blood glucose   Ketones

            mmol/L

                                                  BMI

Ht: Wt: Target Wt:

Allergies   Alcohol

                             Tobacco

Drugs

                             Exercise

Figure 8.2: Diabetes review card format

Occupation				
Family history				
Personal history				
List of educational topics covered				

Figure 8.3: Diabetes review card format (contd.)

Date	BP	URINE			BLOOD GLUCOSE		HbA1$_c$	Foot pulses				Sensation		Vibration	
		G	A	K	mmol/L	hrs post	DP	PT				L	R	L	R
						meal	L R	L	R						

Figure 8.4: Diabetes review card format (contd.)

Visual acuity		Fundi/lens		Results	Notes	Next appt
L	R	L	R	U&Es etc		

Figure 8.5: Diabetes review card format (contd.)

Referral policies

The CSAG (1994) has specified referral to specialist diabetes teams in special situations. Diabetes UK suggested the inclusion of referral criteria in district diabetes management policies and in individual practice policies. Examples of referral criteria were included in national recommendations and guidelines (BDA, 1997b; RCN, 1994).

The CSAG provided broad categories of patients for referral, who either have complications or are at increased risk of complications. Their recommendations placed particular emphasis on the importance of ophthalmological referrals (CSAG, 1994).

Other groups of patients who require specialist input include pregnant women, children and young people (see standard 9 of the NSF). The Royal College of Nursing (1994) suggests the referral of new patients with Type 1 diabetes and Diabetes UK suggested those converting to insulin, although there is a trend for increasing numbers of patients to be converted to insulin in primary care settings. Patients with ketoacidosis require management by hospitals.

Audit

Audit is an evaluation of current practice, in order to introduce change and raise standards. The metaphor of a spiral describes a sequence of audit cycles (Norman, 1995); each cycle to consist of several phases (Figure 8.6).

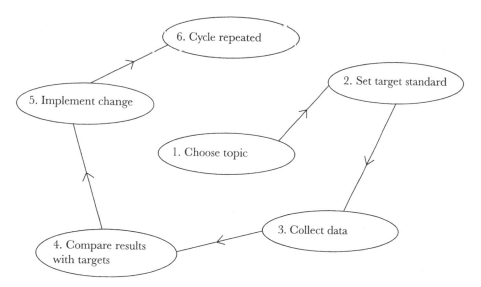

Figure 8.6: An audit spiral

The government response to recommendations in the *Standards of Care for People with Diabetes* required GP practices to carry out clinical audits (CSAG, 1994). A clinical audit is an audit of any aspect of clinical care carried out by the practice team and it can prove to be a satisfying and motivating experience for participants. There are a variety of innovative methods for carrying out audits (Irvine and Irvine, 1991). Audit is not the compilation of a set of statistics relating to practice activities, for inclusion in the practice annual report (metaphorically a linear process in which no actual changes are made).

Diabetes UK suggested that process measures of the quality of diabetes care and measures of the outcomes of care should be used in clinical audit (see Box 8.11).

Box 8.11: Examples of measures for use in clinical audit

Process measures:
- Proportion of patients who have had visual acuity and fundoscopy carried out within the last year
- Proportion of patients who have had their blood pressure measured within the last year

Measures of outcomes of care:
- Proportion of patients who have had laser treatment for diabetic retinopathy
- Proportion of patients with blood pressure of > 140/90

Source: Adapted from BDA (1997b).

Audit criteria should be drawn from expert guidelines. Standards are identified for criteria (for example: 100 per cent of patients will have a fundoscopy carried out each year). Published tables may be used to calculate the sample size (Baker et al., 1993). This ensures the reliability and validity of the audit. Future selection of standards will reflect NSF requirements.

Recent emphasis on the development of quality initiatives within the NHS has prompted the development of national clinical guidelines. It remains to be seen how the quality initiatives outlined in the recent white paper are organized, but audit will remain a vital component (DoH, 1997). Clinical governance meetings offer a forum for clinical review and development. The problem of reconciling PCT and health care trust corporate policies on clinical governance has yet to be resolved.

Professional links

The professional links section of the content requirements schedule required GPs to 'Work together with other professionals when appropriate'. This requisite constituted an acknowledgement of the multi-professional approach to diabetes care in the community that had been developing in Britain since the early 1980s. The emphasis on this approach is continued within standard 12 of the diabetes NSF with a requirement to ensure all people with diabetes requiring multi-agency support receive integrated health and social care (Department of Health, 2001a).

In 1994 the CSAG published a report on standards of care for people with diabetes (see Box 8.12).

Box 8.12: Indicative content list of CSAG recommendations for standards of diabetes care

- The relevance of quality in diabetes health care
- Patient-centred care
- The teamwork approach
- The importance of preventive care
- Internal monitoring of the quality of care
- Guidelines for care
- Diabetes registers and organization of records

Diabetes UK used the title of Local Diabetes Service Advisory Groups (LDSAGs) to refer to the CSAG's proposed local planning groups (BDA, 1994) and produced a response document in 1995 see (see Box 8.13).

Box 8.13: Definition of a Local Diabetes Service Advisory Group

The LDSAG is a group of people with a long-term purpose: to contribute to the formation of a comprehensive local strategy for diabetes management, to advise on and monitor the health care and social services for people with diabetes, to make recommendations and to advise on improvements (clinical and administrative), and to provide a high-quality service to local people with diabetes that meets their needs and wishes.

At that time, 83 out of 154 health authorities had multidisciplinary diabetes advisory groups (BDA, 1995). The NSF for Diabetes Delivery Strategy (DoH, 2003) has suggested that Diabetes Networks be developed, bringing together a range of players, including front-line staff and people with diabetes. These will be directly accountable to PCTs and are likely to replace LDSAGs. The National Health Service Executive published a document that emphasized the need to monitor the quality and effectiveness of diabetes services (National Health Service Executive, 1997). It identified the development of a seamless service, working across primary and secondary health care settings as a main objective. Practice nurses, diabetes nurse specialists, health visitors, community and school nurses are mentioned for inclusion in the consultative process of developing structured programmes of care.

The New NHS: Modern – Dependable included several potential influences for new directions in diabetes care (DoH, 1997). Diabetes UK stressed the important opportunity presented by the inclusion of community nursing representatives in the new Primary Care Groups (PCGs), which assumed responsibility for commissioning local diabetes services (BDA, 1998). Diabetes care is included in health improvement programmes (HimPs) and some districts have identified diabetes as the focus for a local HimP. Since April 2001 Primary Care Trust status has been granted to many of the PCGs, and there has been an increase in the number of specialist nurses employed directly by PCTs. An additional incentive was the pending National Service Framework for diabetes, which would require PCTs to demonstrate the framework and support they provided to achieve acceptable standards of care in all settings.

Description of Nurses employed in the Community

In many districts a nursing adviser was appointed by the District Health Authority to advise on nursing matters. Advisers might have input on matters such as training, employment and funding for nurses. They particularly have an influential role in local practice nursing. More recently PCTs have assumed the role of employers.

Practice nurses

During the last decade, the number of practice nurses has risen dramatically. This rise in numbers has coincided with the increase in the number of general practices running diabetic clinics.

Diabetes care training for practice nurses

In 1993 the General Medical Services Committee (GMSC) stated that: 'any health professionals involved in the care of patients in the programme should be appropriately trained in the management of diabetes' (1993, 9). This statement placed a responsibility on general practitioners as employers of nurses to provide suitable training opportunities for their staff. The National Health Service Executive (1997) also stipulated that there should be a structured programme of continuing education for all health care professionals involved in the service. The GMSC document specified that: 'Training should be matched to the level of involvement in the programmes' (1993: 23).

At the time of writing the final documents for the NSF are not available, but they are likely to include new recommendations about training.

In 1994 the RCN expanded this idea of different levels of involvement when it produced a set of *Diabetes Clinical Guidelines for Practice Nurses*. The document identified minimum, moderate and maximum levels of involvement. It included minimum training requirements, aims and responsibilities at these levels, but did not link these levels of involvement to different levels of pay (RCN, 1994).

The minimum level clinical procedures were intended to be suitable for all practice nurses. The moderate level included a list of educational responsibilities. The maximum level added further educational responsibilities, advising on management of therapy, participation in decisions about care and treatment and a requirement to audit standards of care.

Another definition of the role for practice nurses in GP diabetes clinics was provided by Diabetes UK in the document *Recommendations for the Management of Diabetes in Primary Care* (BDA, 1993).

District (community) nurses

Primary Care Trusts have become the employers of district nurses. District nurses continue to undertake the majority of diabetes care for people who require care either in their own homes or in local authority sheltered accommodation and homes (see Box 8.14).

Box 8.14: Examples of tasks undertaken by district nurses

- Monitoring blood glucose levels
- Drawing up and administering insulin injections
- Management of foot ulcers

They have important responsibilities for the care of people disabled by the complications of diabetes on daily and long-term bases.

The RCN (1994) included a protocol for the commencement of insulin therapy by district nurses. In some practices the district nurses may undertake specified tasks in connection with routine or annual screening reviews.

Nurse practitioners

A few districts have also seen the employment of nurse practitioners by general practices. Moores (1996) defined a nurse practitioner as 'a nurse to whom people have direct access, and who accesses, diagnoses, treats and discharges or refers on to other professional colleagues'. Nurse practitioners undertake a more extensive role in the diagnosis, management of treatment and screening than practice nurses and district nurses. Their functions incline towards medicine rather than traditional nursing.

Diabetes specialist nurses (DSNs) and diabetes specialist health visitors

In some districts diabetes specialist nurses or even health visitors have been employed to offer education and care to patients in the community in order to reduce the number of patients requiring admission to hospital. Both groups of nurses might carry out domiciliary visits, for instance to children with diabetes, and could be involved with commencement of insulin therapy on an outpatient basis. An increasing number are being employed by PCTs.

Diabetes specialist health visitors may, but do not necessarily, have particular responsibilities for working with children and adolescents. In recent years paediatric home care teams have multiplied in number and may include members with diabetes qualifications.

Diabetes facilitators

Diabetes facilitators aim to improve standards of diabetes care in the community. They function as trainers. The employment circumstances of facilitators vary. Some are experienced diabetes nurse specialists; they deliver the specialist content of training sessions themselves and attend clinics. Other facilitators are employed as generic primary health care facilitators and are concerned with diabetes care for either all or some of their working hours (Wilson and Noakes, 1997). The employment of specialist nurses by PCTs is the latest trend, which is likely to include facilitation of general practices.

Care Settings

This section begins with some information on diabetes shared-care schemes; it continues with a review of different care settings within the community.

Shared care

Pritchard and Hughes defined the term 'shared care' (1995: 3) (see Box 8.15).

Box 8.15: Definition of the term 'shared care'

'The responsibility for the health care of the patient is shared between individuals or teams who are part of separate organizations, or where substantial organizational boundaries exist.'

Diabetes care was one of the earliest clinical domains for shared-care schemes. Since 1970 a substantial number of schemes have been established whereby care is shared between general practices and specialist diabetes care teams. Patients may receive an initial assessment and annual reviews from the specialist hospital-based teams and routine reviews from their GP. Pritchard and Hughes (1995) stated that for a shared-care scheme to be effective it must employ a method of information exchange more sophisticated than the traditional referral letter and reply. A patient-held record is one example of a manual system for transferring data between the patient, a general practitioner and a specialist doctor or nurse. This is also perceived as a strategy for empowering patients, endorsed by standard 3 of the National Service Framework. Likewise the NSF cites the development of nationwide information systems using a standard core data set. Initiatives to set up district and nationwide computer-based diabetes information systems are likely to fuel the development of further numbers of shared-care schemes. But the term 'shared care' has also evolved to encompass the concept of partnerships and the use of integrated care pathways (ICPs).

Sole care for people with diabetes may be provided at either their GP's surgery or a hospital. In addition to hospital outpatient departments, diabetes day care centres and elderly day hospitals, diabetes reviews may be carried out in a number of community settings.

GPs' surgeries

General practices organize chronic disease programmes for diabetes in a variety of ways. Some group practices run diabetes 'miniclinics' in blocks of 'protected time', where both the practice nurse and the GP see patients for 20 minutes. Alternatively it may be only the practice nurse who sees patients with diabetes, in a 10-minute appointment which the patient had made for some other reason.

The WHO's St Vincent's Declaration, to which Britain was a signatory, required health care professionals to promote 'equality for elderly people with diabetes' (CSAG, 1994: 40). The next section includes a short synopsis of care provided for elderly and disabled residents and patients in non-NHS institutions.

Patients' own homes

Dornan et al. (1992) found poor life quality and a higher prevalence of dementia and undetected depression amongst elderly people with diabetes in the community compared with their non-diabetic peers. They suggested that the care of the elderly person with diabetes should not be too narrowly focused on metabolic goals.

There appears to be a lack of objective evidence about the proportion of district nurses, nurse practitioners and practice nurses who undertake annual and routine screening for the housebound elderly. Domiciliary care was traditionally the domain of district nurses. It is difficult to find objective evidence that their role has expanded to include more extensive participation in the screening requirements for diabetes chronic disease management programmes.

It is equally difficult to establish that substantial numbers of practice nurses are undertaking home visits. Potentially, nurse practitioners could incorporate this task as part of their role, because of their additional training to undertake physical examinations and diagnoses.

Sheltered housing

Butler et al. (1983) defined sheltered housing as grouped (flats or bungalows) independent accommodation linked to a resident warden by an alarm system.

There are varying degrees of support available to residents according to the degree of independence of the occupants. The role of a warden in diabetes care is likely to be minimal. Wardens may benefit from awareness of the signs and treatment of hypoglycaemia in elderly people, particularly when caring for confused people with diabetes. They may also need to be aware of the risks of ketoacidosis in Type 1 diabetes and know in what circumstances urgent medical help should be summoned. Help may also be available from home helps and district nurses. Each occupant will be dependent on their GP for organizing the provision of diabetes care.

Residential homes

Residential homes are increasingly privately funded, with the role of local authorities shifting from providing places via social services and housing departments, to purchasing by social services departments. A proportion of places continue to be provided by local authorities: 'Part III accommodation' refers to the local authority provision of residential accommodation under the 1948 National Assistance Act. Residents are dependent on staff to carry out the daily activities of living. Residential homes are not required to employ qualified nurses on a 24-hour basis. Diabetes care is thus mainly provided by unqualified health care assistants who may hold NVQ qualifications. Daily monitoring and observations are their main responsibilities and are similar to those undertaken by their counterparts in nursing homes (see Box 8.16). Insulin injections are usually carried out by district nurses.

Box 8.16: The role of care assistants in residential and nursing homes

- Blood or urine glucose monitoring
- Administration of oral hypoglycaemic agents
- Observation and reporting of hypoglycaemic episodes
- Attention to nutritional intake
- Daily foot hygiene and inspection
- Observation for signs of infection

Nursing homes

Nursing homes are required by people who need nursing care in addition to assistance with the daily activities of living. Diabetes UK produced a guide for the staff of residential homes (BDA, 1997c). Gadsby (1994) emphasized the need for staff education in homes.

District nurses are rarely involved in the care of patients in privately owned nursing homes. Registered nurses employed by the homes carry out equivalent tasks.

The GPs who act as medical officers for residential homes will have overall responsibility for ensuring that residents receive an equitable share of diabetes care. Individual GPs would ideally have an agreed procedure with each nursing home for the provision of initial, annual and routine reviews.

Some diabetes care initiatives have been aimed at increasing the expertise of care staff in residential homes, who are the main carers for those residents who have diabetes. Hall (1992), a practice nurse, described her contact with one home that centred on education of staff. She did not, however, address the often neglected issue of the role of nurses in screening these residents for complications.

Gadsby (1994) highlighted a fundamental problem likely to limit the standard of care offered by privately owned nursing homes, which is the minimal number of qualified staff employed in nursing homes. Tong et al. (1994) also expressed concern at their finding that less than half of frail elderly residents included in their audit had received any formal review of their diabetes. They concluded that there had been relatively poor provision of diabetes care to frail elderly residents in residential and nursing homes compared with those living in their own homes.

National Service Framework

The NSF diabetes standards document specifies service models, intervention details and supplementary information. The service models include one on consultation. Within this model there is a section on 'empowering people with diabetes', which is centred on care plans and patient-held/accessed records.

The NSF standards relevant to this chapter are shown in Box 8.17. Strategies in standard 1 include exercise programmes on prescription, weight loss groups, and so on. For standards 5 and 6, communication with clinics is important to ensure patients are not lost to follow-up – particularly at transition from paediatric to adult care. Under standard 7 it is especially important to know when to refer to hospital. Standard 9 should include referral of all pregnant patients for secondary care during their pregnancy, and this should be done at the earliest opportunity. Provision of pre-pregnancy counselling is also important – particularly for women who are irregular attenders at hospital clinics.

Box 8.17: NSF standards

Standard 1: Prevention of Type 2 diabetes

(1) The NHS will develop, implement and monitor strategies to reduce the risk of developing Type 2 diabetes in the population as a whole and to reduce the inequalities in the risk of developing Type 2 diabetes.

Standard 2: Identification of people with diabetes

(2) the NHS will develop, implement and monitor strategies to identify people who do not know they have diabetes.

(contd)

Standard 3: Empowering people with diabetes

(3)   All children, young people and adults with diabetes will receive a service which encourages partnership in decision-making, supports them in managing their diabetes and helps them to adopt and maintain a healthy lifestyle. This will be reflected in an agreed and shared care plan in an appropriate format and language. Where appropriate, parents and carers should be fully engaged in this process.

Standard 4: Clinical care of adults with diabetes

(4)   All adults with diabetes will receive high-quality care throughout their lifetime, including support to optimize the control of their blood glucose, blood pressure and other risk factors for developing the complications of diabetes.

Standards 5 and 6: Clinical care of children and young people with diabetes

(5)   All children and young people with diabetes will receive consistently high-quality care and they, with their families, and others involved in their day-to-day care, will be supported to optimize the control of their blood glucose and their physical, psychological, intellectual, educational and social development.
(6)   All young people with diabetes will experience a smooth transition of care from paediatric diabetes services to adult diabetes services, whether hospital or community based, either directly or via a young people's clinic. The transition will be organized in partnership with each individual and at an age appropriate to and agreed with them.

Standard 7: Management of diabetic emergencies

(7)   the NHS will develop, implement and monitor agreed protocols for rapid and effective treatment of diabetic emergencies by appropriately trained health care professionals. Protocols will include the management of acute complications and procedures to minimize the risk of recurrence.

Standard 9: Diabetes and pregnancy

(9)   The NHS will develop, implement and monitor policies that seek to empower and support women with pre-existing diabetes and those who develop diabetes during pregnancy to optimize the outcome of their pregnancy.

Standards 10, 11 and 12: Detection and management of long-term complications

(10) All young people and adults with diabetes will receive regular surveillance for the long-term complications of diabetes.
(11) The NHS will develop, implement and monitor agreed protocols and systems of care to ensure that all people who develop long-term complications of diabetes receive timely, appropriate and effective investigation and treatment to reduce their risk of disability and premature death.
(12) All people with diabetes requiring multi-agency support will receive integrated health and social care.

Questions (one for each learning outcome)

(1) Mrs Ward is 80 years old and has had Type 2 diabetes for 10 years. She has developed a neuropathic foot ulcer. She has been advised to avoid walking as much as possible in order to reduce pressure on her foot. A recent HbA1$_c$ result was 13 per cent and she has been advised that she needs to improve the control of her diabetes. (a) Which health care professionals might be available to provide the care that she requires as an outpatient? (b) List three alternative options for the provision of screening reviews for her.

(2) Mr Dixon is 86 years old and has had Type 1 diabetes for 20 years. His wife has died and he is unable to look after himself. He has decided to move into residential accommodation. List the types of residential accommodation that he should consider and the people who would assist him with his diabetes care.

(3) Mrs Goel has recently arrived in England to live with her daughter. She is aged 75 and can speak English. Make a list of what care you would tell her to expect to receive each year.

Suggested answers may be found on page 258.

References

Baker R, Khunti K, Lakhani M (1993) Monitoring Diabetes CT2, Appendix 2. Leicester: Eli Lilly National Clinical Audit Centre, Department of General Practice, University of Leicester.

British Diabetic Association (1993) Recommendations for the Management of Diabetes in Primary Care. 1st edn. London: British Diabetic Association.

British Diabetic Association (1994) Cornerstones of an Adequate Standard of Diabetes Care. London: British Diabetic Association.

British Diabetic Association (1995) Guidance on Local Diabetes Services Advisory Groups. London: British Diabetic Association.

British Diabetic Association (1997a) Diabetes Care – What you Should Expect. 90EE. London: British Diabetic Association.

British Diabetic Association (1997b) Recommendations for the Management of Diabetes in Primary Care. 2nd edn. London: British Diabetic Association.

British Diabetic Association (1997c) Diabetes Care Today – A Guide for Residential and Nursing Home Managers and Staff. 9SSS. London: British Diabetic Association.

British Diabetic Association (1998) The white paper: a diabetes perspective. Diabetes Update Spring.

British Hypertension Society (2002) Joint British Societies Coronary Risk Prediction Chart. http://www.hyp.ac.uk/bhs/resources_prediction_chart.htm

Butler A, Oldman C, Greve J (1983) Sheltered Housing for the Elderly: Policy, Practice and the Consumer. London: Allen & Unwin.

Clinical Standards Advisory Group (CSAG) (1994) Standards of Clinical Care for People with Diabetes. London: HMSO.

Coles C (1989) Diabetes education: theories of practice. Practical Diabetes 6(5): 199–202.

Day J, Humphreys D, Alban-Davies H (1987) Problems of comprehensive shared diabetes care. British Medical Journal 294: 1590–2.

Department of Health (1990) National Health Service and Community Care Act. Chapter 19, part 5, Section 62. London: HMSO.

Department of Health (1997) The New NHS: Modern – Dependable. CM3807 EL(97)81. London: HMSO.

Department of Health (2000) Preventing coronary heart disease in high risk patients. In Modern Standards and Service Models: Coronary Heart Disease. London: HMSO.

Department of Health (2001a) National Service Framework for Diabetes. http:// www.doh.gov.uk/nsf/diabetes

Department of Health (2001b) National Service Framework for Diabetes – Standards. http://www.doh.gov.uk/nsf/diabetes/ch2/servicemodels.indec.htm

Department of Health (2003) National Service Framework for Diabetes – Delivery Strategy. London: HMSO.

Donnelly R, Enslie-Smith A, Gardner I, Morris A (2000) Vascular complications of diabetes: ABC of arterial and venous disease. British Medical Journal 320: 1062–6.

Dornan T, Peck G, Dow J, Tattersall R (1992) A community survey of diabetes in the elderly. Diabetic Medicine 9: 860–5.

Feher M (1993) Hypertension in Diabetes Mellitus. London: Martin Dunitz.

Fox C, Pickering A (1995) Diabetes in the Real World. London: Class Publishing.

Gadsby R (1994) Care of people with diabetes who are housebound or in nursing homes and residential homes. Diabetes in General Practice 4: 30–1.

Garg A (1994) Management of dyslipidaemia in IDDM patients. Diabetes Care 17: 224–34

General Medical Services Committee (1993) The New Health Promotion Package. Paragraph 30, Schedule 4. London: British Medical Association.

Gilchrist B, Robertson C, Webb C, Wright S (Eds) (1992) The Textbook of Adult Nursing. In Brunner L, Suddarth D (Eds) Assessment and careof patients with visual disturbances and eye disorders. London: Chapman & Hall.

Hall K (1992) Care of the housebound diabetic. Practice Nurse December: 539–42.

Hillingdon NHS Primary Care Trust (2001) Diabetes guidelines. Unpublished document. Produced by Hillingdon Primary Care Trust, The Hillingdon Diabetes Team Diabeticare, Local Diabetes Services Advisory Group, Hillingdon, London.

Irvine D, Irvine S (1991) Making Sense of Audit. Oxford: Radcliffe Medical Press.

Keen H (1994) Management measures from a working party. Chaired by Professor H. Keen, Guy's Hospital. Reviewed at 'Blood Pressure & Diabetes: Everyone's Concern', 26 May.

Klenerman L, McCabe C, Cogley D, Crerand S, Laing P, White M (1996) Screening for patients at risk of diabetic foot ulceration in a general diabetic clinic. Diabetic Medicine 13(6): 561–3.

Lewis R, Gillam S (Eds) (1999) Transforming Primary Care. London: King's Fund.

MacKinnon M (2001) Providing Diabetes Care in General Practice. 4th edn. London: Class Publishing.

McDowell J, Gordon D (Eds) (1996) Diabetes – Caring for Patients in the Community. London: Churchill Livingstone.

Moores Y (1996) Practice Nurse 8 March.

National Health Service Executive (1997) Key Features of a Good Diabetes Service. Health Service Guidelines HSG(97)45. London: Department of Health.

Norman I (1995) Making a start on clinical audit: cycles and spirals. In Kogan M, Redfern S (Eds) Making use of Clinical Audit. Buckingham: Open University Press.

Patchett P, Roberts D (1994) Diabetic patients who do not have diabetes: investigation of register of diabetic patients in general practice. British Medical Journal 308: 1225–6.

Pritchard P, Hughes J (1995) Shared Care – the Future Imperative. London: The Royal Society of Medicine Press.

Ramsay LE, Williams B, Johnston GD et al (1999) Guidelines for management of hypertension: Report of the Third Working Party of the British Hypertension Society. Journal of Human Hypertension 13(56): 9–92.

Royal College of Nursing (1994) Diabetes Clinical Guidelines for Practice Nurses. Revised edn. London: Royal College of Nursing.

Skinner C (1996) Foot health education. In McDowell J,Gordon D (Eds) Diabetes – Caring for Patients in the Community. London: Churchill Livingstone.

Taylor D, Perkins J (1996) Testing Visual Acuity. Visual Acuity Instruction Chart, Exeter Diabetes and Vascular Centre. London: British Diabetic Association.

Tong P, Baillie S, Roberts S (1994) Diabetes care in the frail elderly. Practical Diabetes 11(4): 163–4.

Wilson Z, Noakes H (1997) Facilitation of diabetes care in general practice. British Journal of Community Nursing 2(2):106–13.

Answers

Chapter 1

(1) The commonest symptoms of Type 2 diabetes are:
- Polyuria and nocturia
- Thirst
- Genital thrush
- Tiredness/weakness
- Blurred vision
- Weight loss

Symptoms such as pruritus and boils may also be an indication of diabetes. Simone also needs to be aware that it is possible to develop diabetes with no or very mild symptoms.

An explanation of why symptoms occur may include the following. If the body is unable to produce enough insulin the sugar (glucose) level in the blood rises and then the sugar spills over into the urine. This leads to an increase in urine production which in turn leads to excessive fluid loss and therefore thirst. The sugar in the urine can cause irritation and thrush, particularly in women. Calories are lost through sugar loss in the urine and therefore some (but not all) people lose weight when blood sugar levels are high. The lens in the eye (not the back of the eye) can temporarily change shape and vision may be blurred. This does get better.

(2) A laboratory fasting or random venous blood glucose should be performed. Michael should be questioned with regard to the symptoms such as thirst, nocturia, tiredness, weight loss, etc. He should also be asked whether anyone in his family has diabetes and which type they have.

A random venous plasma glucose (RBG) of ≥ 11.1 mmol/L plus symptoms or a fasting venous plasma glucose of ≥ 7.0 mmol/L would confirm diagnosis.

If symptoms are not present another venous blood glucose test is required. If results are equivocal an OGTT is required.

(3)
- Test urine (or blood) for ketones
- Family history of diabetes
- Symptoms of diabetes:
  (i) severity
  (ii) duration
- Weight:
  (i) Has it decreased? If yes, by how much and over what period of time?
- Sharon's age
- Bicarbonate result (if available)

The following are strongly suggestive of Type 1 diabetes:
- Urine/blood contains moderate/large ketones despite having eaten
- Severe symptoms of diabetes over a period of weeks (not months or years)
- Weight loss of usually more than half a stone
- Age of 30 years or less
- A lowered venous bicarbonate level

The following are strongly suggestive of Type 2 diabetes:
- Negative or small ketones in urine/blood
- Family member with Type 2 diabetes
- Symptoms of diabetes occurring over a few months
- No weight loss
- 40 years or older (if Caucasian – Type 2 diabetes may occur at a younger age in some races)
- Bicarbonate within normal range

Chapter 2

(1) You may wish to include:
- Avoid sugary food
- Use sweeteners rather than sugar in tea/coffee
- Have diet or sugar-free drinks
- Stop eating honey and use reduced-sugar jams
- Eat three meals a day and try to eat a piece of fruit between meals
- Make starch the biggest part of the meal, e.g. rice/bread/chapattis/pasta, etc.
- Try to eat less fat
- Grill rather than fry
- Try low-fat spreads
- Try semi-skimmed or skimmed milk

(2) It is important to try diet for about 3 months first.

There are six groups of tablets:
(a) sulphonylureas
(b) biguanides
(c) alpha glucosidase inhibitors.
(d) thiazolidinediones
(e) meglitinides
(f) amino acid derivatives

(a) Sulphonylureas, e.g. gliclazide, glibenclamide, work by stimulating insulin production. They are ideal for those who are slim. They have few side-effects, the main ones being hypoglycaemia and possible weight gain. They should be taken before meals.
(b) Biguanides, e.g. metformin, work by helping to stop the liver producing new glucose and help insulin carry glucose into muscle and fat cells more effectively. Ideal for those who are overweight. They do not cause hypoglycaemia if used alone. Main side-effects are diarrhoea and abdominal pain; these are less likely to occur if metformin is introduced gradually and taken after food.
(c) Alpha-glucosidase inhibitors, e.g. acarbose (Glucobay), work by slowing down the absorption of carbohydrates (starchy foods) from the intestine and slow down the rise in blood glucose after meals. They do not cause hypoglycaemia if used alone. If used in conjunction with sulphonylureas, glucose rather than sucrose should be used to treat hypoglycaemia. Acarbose should be chewed with the first mouthful of food. Its main side-effect is wind and the dose should therefore be increased gradually.
(d) Thiazolidinediones, e.g. rosiglitazone, pioglitazone, target insulin resistance, increasing the sensitivity of peripheral tissues to insulin and decreasing the production of glucose by the liver. They must be used in conjunction with either a sulphonylurea or metformin (but not with both together). Liver function tests must be performed every 2 months for at least the first year of treatment. They can lead to fluid retention and are contraindicated in heart failure.
(e) Meglitinides, e.g. repaglinide. If taken shortly before meals this increases insulin secretion during the immediate phase after eating and stops blood glucose rising 1½–2 hours after food. It can cause hypoglycaemia and must be taken three times a day. Repaglinide can be used alone or in combination with metformin.
(f) Amino acid derivatives, e.g. nateglinide. This improves early-phase insulin secretion without inducing the prolonged high levels of insulin in the blood seen with other drugs that increase insulin secretion. If taken without food they stimulate very little insulin release, but with food stimulate a large secretion of insulin. This may prevent weight gain and lessen risk of hypoglycaemia. They are licensed to be used in combination with metformin.

(3) It is important to involve Sam in the decision about which insulin regime would be most suitable. Perhaps ask:
- How is he getting on with injections?
- Can he manage the syringe? Would he prefer a pen?
- Has he had any thoughts of his own about different regimes or spoken to others with diabetes?

The two insulin regimes most likely to be suitable are:
(a) twice a day free-mixed soluble and isophane insulin
(b) basal bolus regime: soluble or analogue insulin pre-meal and isophane before bed.

The benefits and disadvantages of each should be discussed. Then Sam should be encouraged to choose which he prefers, and reassurance should be given that he can change his mind later.

(a) Twice a day free-mixed
Advantages:
- only two injections per day
- often flexible enough
- soluble insulin could be decreased on Sunday mornings prior to football to prevent hypoglycaemia.

Disadvantages:
- three meals a day plus snacks mid-morning, mid-afternoon and before bed are necessary
- it is difficult to adjust insulin for activities during the afternoon.

(b) Basal bolus
Advantages:
- flexible: meals can be delayed and perhaps occasionally missed. A before-bed snack is often unnecessary. Insulin doses can be increased for extra food or decreased for exercise
- attractive pen available to administer insulin.

Disadvantages:
- four injections per day
- will need to inject at work
- needles for pen device not available on prescription.

Chapter 3

(1) Mrs Martin's age and very high level of blood glucose would perhaps alert you to the fact that she may have HONK.

Helpful questions may include:
(a)
- How long has Mrs Martin been feeling thirsty, tired, passing more urine (i.e. days or weeks/months)?

- Have a lot of fizzy sweet drinks been drunk by Mrs Martin?
- Has Mrs Martin lost any weight recently? How much?
- Is there a family history of diabetes? If yes, which type?
- Does Mrs Martin take any 'water tablets' or tablets for her blood pressure?

(b)
- Urine analysis: large amounts of glucose, negative or small amounts of ketones (protein may be present if HONK precipitated by UTI)
- Urgent U&Es and plasma bicarbonate: bicarbonate normal or slightly low (not acidotic), high plasma sodium
- FBC, MSU, swabs, etc., to look for evidence of infection.

(c)
- Hospital admission
- Intravenous insulin and hypotonic saline. Hourly blood glucose measurements and strict fluid balance charts. Subcutaneous insulin to continue for approximately three months.

(d)
- Either diet alone or diet and oral hypoglycaemic drugs.

(2)
- Improve glycaemic control. Aim for HbA1$_c$ of 7 per cent or less (care regarding hypos). Discuss the benefits of this shown by the DCCT.
- Have eyes examined yearly to look for evidence of changes that can be treated.
- Have BP checked to ensure that it is kept within normal limits as this helps to prevent eye and kidney damage.
- Discuss screening for microalbuminuria. If present, ACE inhibitors have been shown to delay or prevent progression to renal failure.
- Ask Katharine if she smokes. If she does, discuss the effects of smoking on kidneys, eyes, nerves and the cardiovascular system. Provide help and support to stop.
- Discuss the beneficial effects of low-fat, low-salt diet and of regular exercise. Lipids should be checked every three years and weight kept within normal limits. Suggest that Katharine see a state-registered dietitian.
- Feet should be checked yearly for signs of ischaemia and neuropathy. Basic footcare advice should be given.

(3)
- Make arrangements to meet Mr Clough specifically to discuss these problems. Ensure privacy and suggest that he brings his wife with him.
- Find out exactly what the 'few difficulties' are. Ask about:
  (a) libido – stress at work, relationship difficulties, diabetes control;
  (b) other medical problems – including drugs taken;
  (c) determine whether partial or complete erectile failure. Erections on waking?
  (d) painful conditions such as thrush?
  (e) alcohol intake, smoking, recreational drugs;
  (f) changes in the shape of his penis.

- Explain that he will need to see the doctor in the diabetes clinic. Briefly explain that there will be a physical examination including blood tests and that psychological questions will be asked.
- Discuss the available treatments and provide literature and contact phone numbers of Diabetes UK and the Impotence Association.
- Treatment may involve:
  - (a) counselling;
  - (b) changes in drug therapy if taking betablockers, for example;
  - (c) correcting any hormonal deficiencies;
  - (d) intracorporeal injections, vacuum devices or semi-rigid rods.

Chapter 4

(1) Telling patients what to do is not enough!
- The information given should relate to the needs of the individual.
- Professionals should begin by evaluating the knowledge that the patient already has.
- Barriers to learning should be identified and addressed and the patient's fears discussed.
- Information should be given in small easily manageable pieces and knowledge that the patient already has should be built on.
- Understanding should be checked regularly before additional information is given.
- Practical demonstrations should be given and time allocated for patients to practise the technique.
- Jargon and complicated words should be avoided.
- Short-term achievable results should be agreed with patients.
- Patients should not be blamed.
- Patient initiative and independence should be encouraged.

(2) What do Sharon and Peter already know about hypos? Do they have any particular concerns or experiences regarding hypoglycaemia?
- Fears or concerns should be addressed and Sharon's and Peter's questions addressed before any information is given.
- Define hypoglycaemia: 'Make four the floor'.
- Discuss the possible symptoms and advise that the patient may not get all of these symptoms and that they may change over time.
- Testing blood glucose is helpful in determining whether Sharon is hypo or not and Peter may wish to learn this technique too.
- The causes of hypos, such as inadequate amounts of carbohydrate, missed or delayed meals, exercise (including active sex), incorrect timing of injections, alcohol and the honeymoon period, should be explained.
- How hypos can be prevented should be discussed.
- Treatment should be addressed in detail and Sharon and Peter should be provided with glucose tablets, Hypostop and Glucagon. The importance of

eating a high-fibre snack after the symptoms have resolved should be high-lighted.

- If hypos occur, insulin doses may require adjustment. Sharon should be advised to contact the DSN for help and advice as necessary.

(3)
- Establish whether Mr Batty has ever performed testing. If so, which type and why did he stop?
- Discuss the benefits of testing for Mr Batty. These include helping him to regain control over his life. Testing can help him to assess the effects of different foods and activities on his diabetes control.
- Discuss the benefits and disadvantages of urine and blood testing.

Important considerations include:
- Mr Batty is not prone to hypoglycaemia.
- Renal threshold.
- Urine testing is painless and easy to perform.
- Blood testing offers a direct rather than indirect measurement of blood glucose.

Chapter 5

(1) Illness

(a) Answers should include:

- Continue to take gliclazide.
- If cough mixture or cold remedies are taken they should be sugar free.
- Test urine 2–4 times per day.
- If urine tests continue to be 2 per cent consider increasing gliclazide to a maximum of 160 mg bd.
- Continue with usual meals even if urine glucose levels are high.
- Maintain adequate fluid intake.

(b)
- Take all insulin doses although not eating normally.
- Replace usual meals with liquid CHO.
- Test blood for glucose four times per day.
- If blood glucose is 13 mmol/L or more insulin doses should be increased according to protocol.
- Test urine or blood for ketones at least twice a day.

If Sian is unable to tolerate at least one glass of sugary liquid, is vomiting, her blood glucose levels remain high, or ketone tests are moderate or large despite treatment, hospital assessment is necessary.

(2) Travel
- Insulin should be transported in her hand luggage and stored either in a fridge or kept below 25°C.

- Do not aim for 'perfect' control whilst travelling.
- The day will be longer on the outward journey. Additional insulin dosage will therefore be necessary. Kathy may need to contact a DSN or doctor for specific advice on insulin adjustment if she has not travelled across time zones previously.
- Double the quantities of supplies actually needed should be taken.
- Supplies should include: insulin, blood glucose and ketone testing kits, a needle clipper, an ID card, a customs letter, CHO-containing foods and glucose tablets, Lucozade, Hypostop and Glucagon.

(3) Exercise
- Encourage them.

Peter:
- Hypoglycaemia is unlikey, metformin, can be continued and regular CHO should be continued but not increased.

Andrea:
- Blood glucose control should be good before an exercise programme is commenced.
- Blood glucose should be monitored before, during and after exercise. Refined CHO should be taken if blood glucose is low.
- Regular CHO should be taken even if the blood glucose is high; blood glucose levels can fall dramatically hours after exercise.
- The doses of Actrapid should be reduced before the exercise.

Chapter 6

(1)
- Yes. Mr Alexander needs insulin (see Table 6.1).
- Assess ability to draw up and administer insulin safely. Can he see a syringe? Does he prefer a pen? Will he remember to take it? Would he like a district nurse to visit and help him? Involve Mr Alexander in decision-making.
- Identify the level of control necessary to relieve symptoms versus the risks of hypoglycaemia.
- Does he live alone? Has he got a telephone? (This may be relevant regarding nocturnal hypoglycaemia and contact with DSN.)
- Education of friends/neighbours/relatives.

(2)
- Has she a family member whom she would like to interpret for her or would she prefer a hospital interpreter to be arranged?
- What does she already know about diabetes? It is likely that someone else in her family will have Type 2 diabetes.
- What does she usually eat? Has her diet changed since diagnosis? Who does the cooking?
- Her weight: is it increasing or decreasing?

- Does she exercise?
- Symptoms of hyperglycaemia: Is she thirsty, etc.?
- Her health care beliefs: whether she believes that her actions can make a difference. If not, consider introducing her to another woman from her culture who has experienced that it can.

Advice:

- Answer Mrs Patel's questions, challenge any misconceptions or erroneous advice already given.
- Diet as necessary to encourage a low-sugar, high-fibre-containing carbohydrate, low-fat, low-salt diet.
- Teach home urine testing for glucose.
- Encourage exercise, perhaps swimming.

(3)

This will obviously depend on Helen's specific concerns/questions and the information may be given over several visits.

- Ask Helen what particularly concerns her and what information she has already been given.
- It is most likely that she will have a healthy baby.
- It is very unlikely that the baby will have diabetes.
- It is important to plan pregnancy in order to achieve good glycaemic control (confirmed by a normal $HbA1_c$). This has been shown to reduce the risk of abnormalities and big babies.
- She should take folic acid 5 mg prior to and during the first 12–13 weeks of pregnancy.

(4)

(a)

- Stop metformin five to seven days prior to surgery. If blood glucose increases, the gliclazide may need to be increased to maximum dose of 160 mg bd.
- Stop tablets on the morning of the operation. Restart usual tablets with the first meal. Test blood glucose levels on the morning of the operation, postoperatively and 6-hourly thereafter.

(b)

- Convert to insulin before admission for surgery.
- Manage as for case-study 6.1.
- Treat with insulin for at least 2–3 months post-operatively with DSN support and perhaps long-term if the poor control prior to surgery was not due to a potentially solvable cause such as poor diet.

Chapter 7

(1) Specific psychological implications may include:
   (a) fear of hypoglycaemia;
   (b) discrimination and restrictions on lifestyle, e.g. loss of, or need to change

job/career, driving restrictions;

(c) difficulties in achieving the necessary behavioural changes, e.g. diet;

(d) needle phobias, e.g. insulin, blood tests;

(e) fear of long-term diabetic complications;

(f) fear of congenital abnormalities or late stillbirth in a child of a mother with diabetes;

(g) fear of passing on diabetes to the next generation;

(h) negative effects on self-esteem and self-confidence.

(2) Strategies to support patient empowerment include:

- Provide the necessary education and effectively teach the practical skills necessary to allow patients to make informed decisions and work in partnership with professionals.
- Show respect for and acceptance of patient opinions and trust them.
- Ensure that there are no power or status barriers, wherever possible, i.e. coffee drinking, etc.
- No interruptions, ensure privacy.
- Be genuine, honest and consistent.
- Demonstrate unconditional personal regard. Respect patients by listening to them.
- Be empathetic, listen to what is said and be alert to what is not said, tentatively summarizing the basic message.
- Provide reassurance. Give clear explanations and behave in a confident manner.
- Negotiate goals with the patient and acknowledge the patient's responsibility for his or her health.

(3)

Health professional (HP): 'Hello, Jessica, it is good to see you again. Perhaps you would like to talk with me today?' (Open invitation to talk)

Jessica: 'Well yeah, I've not been doing any testing.'

HP: 'Can you tell me a bit more about not testing?' (Open question)

Jessica: 'I just can't bring myself to prick my finger.'

HP: 'You can't bring yourself to do it...' (Verbal following)

(The professional gives Jessica the opportunity to further develop the problem.)

Jessica: 'Yeah – I guess, I don't want to do it. It's not that I can't do it, I know how to do it and why I should.'

HP: 'Perhaps you could tell me more about how you feel?' (Minimal encourager)

Jessica: 'I don't see why I should have to test, I'm only 20 [years old], I shouldn't have to worry about diabetes, I don't want diabetes.'

HP: 'You are worried about diabetes?' (Reflecting feelings)

Jessica: 'I don't like being different and I'm scared I'll get complications. Testing my blood and coming to clinic reminds me that I have diabetes and I don't want to think about it.'

This approach is more likely to be successful than a more traditional medical approach. Typical traditional approaches might include: 'It is important to test your blood in order to adjust your insulin, improve your control and avoid complications'; ' Shall I go over the technique again?'; or 'Why not?' with the standard 'I'm sorry' response. The use of counselling skills identified the problems. Jessica has not yet come to terms with the diagnosis of diabetes and fears complications. These feelings can be acknowledged (concreteness) and clarified (summarization). Goals can then be negotiated to begin to tackle the problems.

Chapter 8

(1)

(a)

- District nurse to assess her needs; inspection of feet to include pedal pulses, sensation; monitor blood glucose levels and dress ulcer.
- Domiciliary visit from a podiatrist to assess and treat her feet.
- Practice nurse, nurse practitioner, district nurse or GP to carry out an initial/routine or annual review of her diabetes.
- Diabetes specialist nurse/health visitor or district nurse to convert her to insulin at home, or transport to take her to the local Diabetes Day Care Centre for a few days for conversion to insulin.

(b)

- Sole care by GP, shared care between GP and diabetes specialist team, sole care of diabetes specialist team.

(2)

- Private residential home, Local Authority (Part III) home, warden-controlled flat or bungalow.
- Warden, health care assistants, practice nurse, nurse practitioner, district nurse, GP, podiatrist.

(3)

- Negotiation of a personal care plan.
- Referral to hospital diabetic clinic for review if appropriate.
- Educational review.
- Recall to surgery for annual and routine reviews with option for review to be carried out at home.
- Review of risk factors: smoking history, alcohol intake, diet, exercise, current medication.
- Clinical tests and examination to assess glycaemic control, renal function, cholesterol, feet, eyes, blood pressure, visual acuity, fundoscopy, weight, reflexes.

Appendix 1

Drawing up a single type of insulin

(1) Wash and dry hands.

(2) Check that the type of insulin is correct and that it is within the expiry date.

(3) Gently tip or rotate the bottle of insulin to ensure that the suspension of insulin is properly mixed. DO NOT shake.

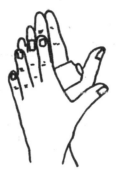

(4) Pull back the plunger to allow the amount of air equivalent to the amount of insulin required to enter the syringe.

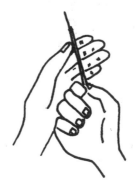

(5) Keeping the bottle cap uppermost, insert the needle through the rubber cap and inject the air into the bottle (this makes it easier to draw up insulin from the bottle).

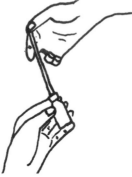

(6) Turn the bottle upside down. Making sure that the point of the needle inside the bottle is covered with fluid, pull back the plunger until slightly more insulin than is required is withdrawn.

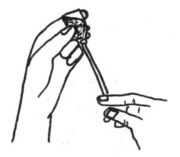

(7) If air bubbles are present gently flick or tap the syringe. When the bubble(s) reach the top of the syringe push the plunger up to expel the air back into the bottle. Expel any surplus insulin back into the bottle.

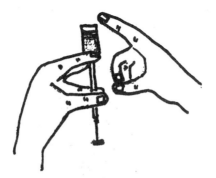

(8) Check that the drawn up dose is correct and then remove the syringe from the bottle.

Appendix 2

Mixing two types of insulin

(1) Wash and dry hands.
(2) Check that the types of insulin are correct and that they are within the expiry date.
(3) Gently tip or rotate the bottles of insulin to ensure that the insulin suspension is properly mixed (this is particularly important with the cloudy insulin). DO NOT shake.

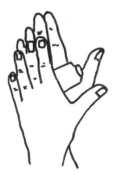

(4) Pull back the syringe plunger to allow the amount of air equivalent to the amount of cloudy insulin required to enter the syringe.

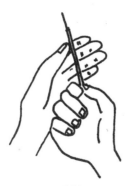

(5) Keeping the bottle cap uppermost, insert the needle through the rubber cap and inject the air into the cloudy insulin bottle.

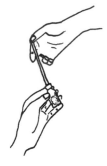

(6) Remove the needle from the bottle.
(7) Pull back the plunger to allow the amount of air equivalent to the amount of clear insulin to enter the syringe.

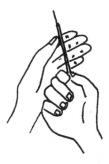

(8) Keeping the bottle cap uppermost insert the needle through the rubber cap and inject the air into the *clear* insulin bottle.

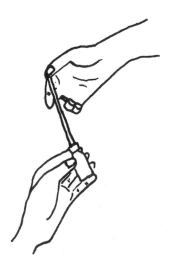

(9) Turn the bottle upside down. Making sure that the point of the needle inside the bottle is covered with *clear* insulin, pull back the plunger until slightly more insulin than is required is withdrawn.

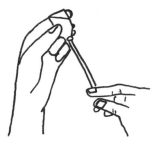

(10) If air bubbles are present flick or tap the syringe. Depress plunger and expel air and any surplus insulin back into the bottle of *clear* insulin.

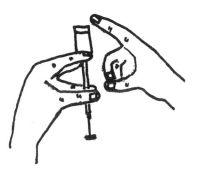

(11) Ensure that the dose of *clear* insulin is correct and then remove from the bottle.
(12) With the bottle turned upside down, carefully insert the needle through the rubber cap of the *cloudy* insulin bottle ensuring that the point of the needle inside the bottle is covered with fluid. Slowly pull back the plunger to the exact dose of *cloudy* insulin. This will then make up the total dose of insulin required, e.g. clear 12 units + cloudy 18 units = total of 30 units.

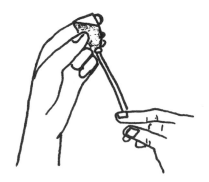

If more cloudy insulin than is required enters the syringe DO NOT expel insulin back into the bottle. The insulins will be mixed and if inserted back into the bottle will contaminate the remaining insulin in the bottle. Expel all the insulin in the syringe down the sink and start again!

(13)   Remove the syringe from the bottle of *cloudy* insulin.

Appendix 3

NSF Diabetes Standards

Topic	Standard number
Prevention of Type 2 diabetes	1
Identification of people with diabetes	2
Empowering people with diabetes	3
Clinical care of adults with diabetes	4
Clinical care of children and young people with diabetes	5, 6
Management of diabetic emergencies	7
Care of people with diabetes during admission to hospital	8
Diabetes and pregnancy	9
Detection and management of long-term complications	10, 11, 12

Source: Adapted from http://www.doh.gov.uk/nsf/diabetes/ch1/standardstable.htm (accessed 06/01/2002).

Index